AN END TO
AGEING?

AN END TO
AGEING?

REMEDIES FOR
LIFE EXTENSION

Stephen Fulder, PhD.

Doctor of Pharmacology and Gerontologist

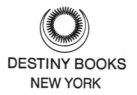

DESTINY BOOKS
NEW YORK

Destiny Books
377 Park Avenue South
New York, New York 10016

U.K. edition published by Thorsons Publishers, Ltd.
Denington Estate, Wellingborough
Northamptonshire, NN8 2RQ England

LIBRARY OF CONGRESS CATALOGING IN PUBLICATION DATA

Fulder, Stephen.
    An end to ageing.
    Bibliography: p.
    1. Ageing. 2. Longevity 3. Health. 4. Herbs—
Therapeutic use. I. Title.
QP86.F84   613   82-5101
ISBN 0-89281-044-0   AACR2

Destiny Books is a division of Inner Traditions International, Ltd.

Printed in the United States of America

CONTENTS

INTRODUCTION

I am a gerontologist by training. This does not mean that I can treat anybody. Gerontology is the study of the process of ageing. It is quite theoretical and biological. Inevitably this approach colours whatever I write on the subject of health and the lifespan. However, when I observe the expanding deluge of health manuals and guidebooks which have appeared over the last few years, it seems that there is an excess of advice and an insufficiency of discussion. A conceptual approach might help people develop a more sophisticated understanding of their health. The guidebooks can then be used more effectively.

During the last few years it has become clearer and clearer to me that the effects of ageing can be modified so that most of us could arrive at old age skipping rather than crawling. This book sets out some ideas and materials which could contribute to this goal. It is an attempt to focus on a few selected possibilities, and is by no means a compendium of methods. Indeed, almost everyone has his own theory on longevity and all this book can provide is some further ammunition. It leans heavily on ginseng as a useful remedy because I happen to have investigated ginseng in the laboratory, and because it appears to be a prime example of the kind of remedy that is relevant to the goal of a healthy old age. There are others, however, and many which are not mentioned in this book.

Health is relative. Health in old age is simply the distillation, the dénouement, of health during the rest of the lifespan. We must all find our own way to a healthy old age by applying the principles that appeal to us as early as possible in our lives. It is the purpose of this book to set the ball rolling.

1
TOWARDS HEALTH IN OLD AGE

An enterprising medical student at Birmingham University recently sat down to some socio-medical research. He collected information on the lifespans of 218 Renaissance artists from a review culled from contemporary sources. He found that this group lived to sixty-seven years. This is a respectable lifespan by any standards, coming close to modern man's expectation of life. Now it is true that this group is especially chosen. They are the ones that made it into history books: a select group of elite individuals well looked after by themselves and society.

Yet it is interesting that despite a risky life full of disease, and in the absence of any sophisticated medicine, this select group managed to live to a ripe old age. How did they manage it? Can we do any better today? Does medicine help us attain our potential lifespan, or does it merely take us safely to maturity and then leave us to an infirm old age?

There are, today, great obstacles in the way of anyone who seeks to attain a healthy long life. Diseases of old age appear as a result of habits, experiences and stresses that accumulate daily. Anyone choosing improved methods of living, whether dietary, physical or psychological is running against a strong current of opinion which refuses to see that life in the West is mostly aggressive, tense, polluted and unhealthy. The struggle for survival in the modern world is fought with the nerves not the muscles, and this kind of struggle has subtle and invisible effects. We do not see people being eaten by sabre-toothed tigers, or falling off cliffs as they must have done in prehistoric times. Instead, we see apparently healthy people engaged in a struggle which in old age brings on such degenerative diseases as arteriosclerosis, coronary failure, and cancer.

When old age arrives the discordant lifestyle continues, for the elderly are not treated with the dignity they need in our western world. Of course we must be thankful that conditions are not so tough that the elderly are despatched as they were by the Eskimos, the Hopi indians or the Bushmen, although even here it was often with ceremony and a paradoxical love that they were consigned to the 'other world'. Yet many peoples give the old a great deal of respect and honour, as, for example, the Zapoteks of Mexico. This tribe lives in extended family units, with each family member, from the oldest to the youngest taking on some of the responsibility. As an ageing adult's abilities decline the rest of the family expect less from him. Thus the old fulfil the role asked of them and do not experience the frustration and stress at failing the community. The old are encouraged to take on necessary chores such as grinding food or caring for children and 'a woman would be happy at ninety provided she is not sick' as one villager stated. The contentment in old age, generated by a sense of harmony within the community, is vital to good health.

Social Isolation – a Blessing in Disguise?

In our culture the aged are hindered at all levels from attaining this state of harmony. Enforced retirement means that those who want to continue the rhythm of a working life are thrust into a crushing slothfulness. They are ensured a loss of respect from a world which judges a person by employment status. Western life is restless, and the old, unless they be politicians or otherwise famous, are neither heeded nor given responsibility. The aged respond to society's low expectation of them by drying up still further, losing their confidence and with it their wealth of experience. This vicious circle is made complete by infirmity which is both a result of, and a cause of, their rejection. Even Jonathan Swift felt this state:

> I awake in such a state of indifference to anything that may happen to the world and in my own narrow circle that I should certainly stay in bed all day if decency and the fear of illness did not arouse me out of it.

The old have been placed in a pointless fringe world outside society. Social welfare is impersonal and only accentuates their impotent dependence. This alienation is hard for those who look back over their shoulders and feel excluded from the things that concern everybody else. On the other hand alienation could be a blessing because it releases a person from the petty problems of the social environment. It could actually be a time of freedom and liberation.

When life's duties are completed and a family raised, there is nothing more to do than give oneself to quiet contemplation of hobbies, things of the moment, or the world of spirit. In many Eastern cultures, the last portion of the lifespan is the time to devote oneself to achieving inner liberation and to prepare to pass on. Unfortunately, there is little sign of this sensible practice in the West. A catalyst is needed to turn social isolation from a curse into a blessing. Banishment is a delight if the exile is in a Garden of Eden. The most important factor is therefore the boat that will transport our elderly traveller peacefully into his pleasant detachment. This boat is, we might say, calm vitality.

The Need for Vitality

Our goal could reasonably be to help the aged attain that extra vitality to break out of their vicious circle. But where is this extra energy and positivity to come from? How can old people, tired and listless, be suddenly made to jump up and find a useful and worthwhile occupation for mind and body? How can one administer a gentle but firm push out of the armchair, to change despondency and negativity into their opposites? It is a momentous problem, and it is made more difficult by the fact that any suggested systems or preparations will have to overcome several obstacles. Firstly, they cannot require a great deal of energy and discipline for that is exactly what is lacking. This mitigates against onerous exercise regimes, meditation or difficult and complex diets. Such instructions can be given to the elderly but few folk will have the stamina to maintain them.

Secondly they must be acceptable to those already in institutional care of one sort or another, or bedridden. Finally they must be effective despite a life time of bad contrary habits.

This is the greatest problem of them all.

The Role of Medicine

It is obvious that for the purposes of attaining a healthy and energetic old age your doctor is an important figure. But he is as much a hindrance as a help. He is a friend in need when you break a bone or incur an acute and life-threatening disease. But he is worse than useless if you desire assistance in attaining more energy, more resistance, more purpose and more years. Consultation with your doctor on these questions would, at best, produce no useful result. At worst, it would generate a reflex response towards the prescription pad to give you toxic medicines (such as anti-depressive or anti-anxiety drugs) which would prevent the very vitality you sought.

The reason for this is that our medical system is designed to get you to old age but is not concerned with the state in which you arrive there. While infant mortality in our culture is very low, and disease of childhood and adulthood are dealt with by vaccinations, treatment and sanitation, after middle age the disease load increases dramatically. Cancer, cardiovascular deteriorations such as arteriosclerosis, thrombosis and coronary heart disease, bronchial problems, renal disease, and so on are extremely widespread, reaching epidemic proportions in some cases. These are the 'degenerative' diseases of later life and they are extremely difficult to treat by medical means. They take quite some time to develop, that is, they have their origin in the earlier parts of the lifespan and reach fruition during later life. They are thus preventable by health-oriented actions taken during the major part of the lifespan before irreversible full-blown disease sets in. Unlike traditional and alternative medical systems, modern medicine is exclusively curative. Which means it is unable to treat conditions of poor health and vitality before they become expressed as irreversible problems in later life.

Surely, it might be argued, the average lifespan has increased dramatically this century as a result of the rise of medicine. Does this not indicate the ability of medicine to give us a long life? It is true that without modern medicine life would be much more of a battle against sickness, we would be expected to suffer more pain, and every ague, plague, pox and boil

would be more dangerous. Think of surgery without anaes-
thetics, pneumonia without antibiotics, diabetes without
insulin.

On the other hand, careful research has shown that much of
the increase in lifespan that has occurred in the last 100 years
has come as a result of public health measures and not
medicines. For example, drains and sanitation introduced in
Victorian times by an administration alarmed at the dramatic
deaths of thousands in the last cholera outbreaks, had the
unexpected additional consequence of reducing tuberculosis.
Drugs came after the event. The flushing toilet, inspection of
cows, and other similar arrangements made greater contri-
butions to longevity than the subsequent pharmaceutical
revolution. There is reliable data showing that those who do
reach a ripe old age are likely to have had very little prior
contact with doctors.

Modern medicine cannot guarantee a ripe old age. We can
only say that medicine when combined with public health
allows *most* people to reach beyond maturity. But at what cost?
The cost is that although most of us reach old age, we arrive in
such a shoddy patched-up state that it is a misery to be there.
The damage is done from birth onwards, as I learnt when I
consulted a doctor about a sore throat in my five month old
daughter. I received enough antibiotics to sterilize a cess-pool.
She recovered spontaneously the next day, gaining valuable
resistance in the process, while I consigned the expensive
chemicals to the dustbin. There are valuable uses for such
substances but this was not one of them.

The damage of curative medicine is that it is too much, too
late. The disease must produce gross recognizable symptoms
before treatment is offered. The doctor cannot tell if you are
going to get arthritis, only if you already have it. The treatment
itself is then strong and drastic although couched in seemingly
innocuous medical language. During treatment harm is done
by not treating the underlying causes of disease, and by letting
a state of 'not-ill-not-well' continue daily. The end result may
be an unhealthy old age.

For these reasons we will be discussing ideas and remedies
that are largely outside conventional medicine and outside
pathology. We will be looking at herbal 'anti-ageing' remedies,
particularly ginseng, which are important in traditional or folk

medicine. There are indeed medical systems, particularly Far Eastern, which include a good deal of specific instruction on attaining a healthy old age, and some material will be included from these sources. It is not our intention, however, to list all relevant folk remedies and recommend the reader to take them. Medicinal plants should only be taken as part of a therapy. Indiscriminate dabbling in potions is not recommended.

Health is an individual matter and the best advice should be personal, tailor-made to each individual's strengths, weaknesses, lifestyle and constitution. Since most members of the medical profession will be unable to guide an individual towards maximal vitality in old age, practitioners using traditional and subtle health skills must be consulted. Having found such a guide, it would be appropriate to discuss some of the ideas raised in this book with him or her. The development of personal health regimes is discussed in the final chapter.

2
AGEING

There are so many ways in which the human body can fail during ageing that it is impossible to define ageing in any thoroughly specific manner. One can only say that ageing is a progressive increase in susceptibility to an ever greater number of harmful or pathological events. The body is overwhelmed by damage and grinds slowly to a halt.

All living things age. This is not such an easy statement to make and it is disputed. There would be no dispute about mammals which age before our eyes, with wrinkled skin, white hair, clogged blood vessels, slowness and weakness, and those features we know so well from looking at old people. There are arguments about fish however. Sturgeon ringed by the Tsarist household over three hundred years ago have been reportedly found in Russia and the fish seem to continue growing, be it ever more slowly. However, they show age-changes and die in the end, as do certain tortoises and other long-lived amphibia. The oldest living things are trees, the bristlecone pines of California, the oldest of which are known to have lived for more than four thousand years. Their dead bark, like our skin, is continually replenished by a layer of living tissue. This tissue is indeed very old, and may be regarded as almost immortal. So too may be organisms which reproduce by perpetual budding – sea anemones, amoeba, bacteria and other primitive creatures.

However, before ascribing to these primaeval forms an

immortality lost to us, let us look closer at them. If we do this we find that individual cells are ageing and dying, but the community of cells continues indefinitely. To ascribe immortality to them is like a spaceman viewing the teeming Earth and thinking that humans are immortal because they are always there. Immortality does not exist. It cannot exist because if it did there would be no change or development. No new forms of life would emerge. Change is the essence of life and in this sense immortality, paradoxically, is death!

The Human Lifespan

Stories grow longer in the telling. Lifespans also. The further back we travel into mythological time the greater the lifespans our ancestors seem to have been blessed with. Moses lived to 120, Methusaleh to 969, and Noah to 950. 'First men', whether Hindu or Biblical, are sometimes held to be immortal, at least before their 'Fall'.

Scientific investigation, far from confirming the wonderful staying power of our forbears, has indicated exactly the opposite; that the further back we look, the shorter was the human lifespan, and the life expectancy today is longer than it has ever been. The ancient ones seem to be so old only because man is *laudator temporis acti* – he worships ancient times. Today man would not hunger so much for those halcyon days if he was aware that perhaps one baby in three reached adulthood, that death was just as likely at 30 as at 70 and that any minor incident or accident, such as a sore throat, could have fatal consequences.

We know of this by examining skeletons of prehistoric man. Close analysis of the skeletons at different ages tells us that the stages in man's development from birth to maturity are similar in a stone age or a modern man. Yet in neanderthal man, none of the skeletons are older than 40, and in neolithic times none are older than 50. They died from accidents, infections, battles and plagues. In the early written history of the Egyptians, Greeks and Hebrews we do not see a great improvement in *average* lifespan; roughly 75 per cent died before 50 and less than 20 per cent of the population lived beyond 60. In America before the white man arrived the Indians did a bit better; 50 per cent were dead before 50 and

25 per cent lived beyond 60. The chances of dying were more or less the same at any age. It is only when we come to Europe in the eighteenth century that the number of aged people increases. By the mid-nineteenth century, 40 per cent lived beyond 60, in 1900 it was about 50 per cent and now it is about 77 per cent.

Today the life expectancy in the Western world is about 72 years. Since deaths at all ages, even in infancy, are incorporated into the figure of life expectancy, it is an average: an expectation not a goal. The potential of maximum human lifespan is still greater than this. It is not unrealistic to imagine a utopia where we would all be healthy until our maximum lifespan, say a round century, and then drop dead painlessly and diseaselessly from old age. However, this utopia is still a long way away. From 1900 to 1950 the life expectancy increased by 19 years. From 1950 until today the gain has only been 2.4 years and since 1970 it has been 1 year, and that despite an annual spending on medical research that is nothing short of collossal. While medical and social advances in the last 100 years have narrowed the gap between the average and the potential lifespan, progress has now ground to a halt.

Life Stages

The physicians under Hippocrates, nearly two-and-a-half millenia ago introduced a fourfold division of the lifespan which corresponded to the essences of man: childhood (hot and moist), youth (hot and dry), adulthood (cold and moist) and old age (cold and dry). There have been a great number of suggestions as to the beginning of old age. Hippocrates thought it began at 42, and today most agree that it is somewhere between 40 and 50. Such considerations are, however, fruitless, for we have seen that ageing does not pay attention to the calendar. At every point in the lifespan there are irreversible changes which flow gradually one into the other. Conception leads to development, to birth, to growing up, to puberty, to peak vigour, to adulthood and beyond. One can indeed justify the view that ageing begins in a subtle manner the moment the sperm and egg unite and the changes begin to unfold.

Yet when a man is confronting his own ageing it is of little comfort to know that his body has always been ageing. Instead he needs to see the milestones passed and those to come. For him the greatest comfort can be had from traditional views which are psychological and social rather than biological. The Vedas, for example, also point to four stages. The first stage is youth and learning, followed by adulthood and family raising, then a stage of learning, experience and preparation for old age, and finally the stage when it is the time to be released from social duties and family ties, and devote oneself to a life of relaxation and contemplation. Old age becomes, then, a time of release towards which individuals sometimes look with longing. By way of contrast, the life stages in modern America appear to be shocked and helpless tra.isitions. According to *Passages* a study by G. Sheehy, there are seven stages in the American Lifespan, each one usually preceded by psychological and emotional crises.

Sex and Ageing

The most serious of the lifespan crises is often associated with the menopause. The decline in sexual vitality and the menopause are partly the result of changes in the manufacture of hormones. However, the severity of menopausal symptoms is related to the background of general health of mind and body against which the hormone change occurs.

The ovary is the first organ to degenerate with age. It begins to decline in weight at thirty, and the stock of eggs (ova) in the ovary thereafter rapidly becomes exhausted. As the ovary runs out of eggs, its ability to make the female sex hormone, oestrogen, follows suit. The brain pours out other hormone signals to the ovaries, to attempt to restore oestrogen, but the ovaries cannot respond. While the fertility changes are the result of a drop in oestrogen, the depressions and discomforts of the menopause are the result of compensatory changes. The normal but unpleasant side-effects of the menopause may be hot flushes, chills, sweats and headaches, dizziness, depression or irritability, aches in joints and bones, diabetes, muscular weakness and changing skin texture. Since hormones pace the menopause, and hormones are to some extent under our control, the menopause is known to be hastened by stress factors such as overwork or bad health. The symptoms of the menopause are to some extent also influenced by attitude, mood and personality. A negative attitude accentuates them, and a positive vital intention reduces them.

Men do not experience such a precipitous change in fertility and sexual vigour, probably because the testes do not run out of sperm or hormone manufacturing capacity. Nevertheless, there is often a type of discomfiting male menopause due to a partial decline in the male sex hormone testosterone. Men are also not so fortunate to miss a menopause for their hormone patterns appear to make them more vulnerable than women to heart diseases.

Sexual activity and fertility declines with age, particularly in relation to the frequency of intercourse, and the intensity of the experience, yet it need be no less joyful. An erection is harder to obtain but can be maintained for longer. In America, sexologists have reported that the mean age for ceasing intercourse is 68 in married men and 58 in unmarried men. This means that a large proportion of American couples are still sexually active in their sixties with some continuing into their eighties. Regular coitus to mutual orgasm was reported in one man aged 103 and his 90-year-old wife. Naturally those Chinese who make an art of longevity practices expect to be fertile and virile into very old age.

How does sexual activity affect ageing? This has been a subject of unremitting fascination to those interested in health. It used to be assumed that continence lengthened male life because it prevented 'wastage' of sperm or sexual fluids. A little thought would reveal something wrong in this reasoning. Do you gain health by conserving muscular strength? Body organs atrophy with non-use, and become active and efficient with use. The concept of wastage arises from the analogy that the body works like a machine that stays new if you don't use it. The theory may also have been a puritanical self-justification. Medical research shows that moderate practice contributes to the health and function of the sexual organs and has a salutary effect on the health of the body as a whole; continuing sexual activity lengthens life. For example married people live on average longer than unmarried. While the mortality (overall death rate) of Anglican clergymen was found to be only 69 per cent of general male mortality, that of the celibate Roman

Catholic clergy was greater by 5 per cent. It is well known that regular mating improves the condition and the longevity of male agricultural animals.

Naturally, it would be foolish to indulge in excesses sexually as well as in other applications of human energy. As we shall see, the key to successful ageing seems to lie in walking a narrow line between moderation and quiescence on the one hand, and regular practice on the other. This certainly applies to sexual activity. In human society sex is interwoven with the lifespan in myths and the human psychological archetypes. The control or use of sexual activity plays a significant part in traditional systems of knowledge on lengthening life.

Disease and Ageing

We all age at different rates and in different ways. An aborigine will age differently from a businessman, a businessman from his friend and even from his twin brother. One person can have diabetes, white hair or cancer at 30, another none of these at 90. When it is necessary to measure the age of the body, in body-time not clock-time, doctors can usually only use the kind of inspired guesswork of the fairground age-forecaster.

Alex Comfort, realizing the impossibility of measuring ageing by any one of its diverse results, suggested that measurement be made of a multitude of diverse changes. The results could be fed into a computer to get an overall measurement. Included in this were psychological, physiological, anthropometric, biochemical and optometric tests. This has been done, and the procedure is quite useful. It has told us, for example, that radiation has been found to increase the rate of ageing while cigarettes, although they may cause cancer, do not hasten the rate of ageing.

Ageing is not a disease. One can age without disease, however, as ageing progresses the body becomes more vulnerable. Therefore disease is only a symptom or a result of ageing, like white hair, a weak heart, chilblains, tiredness, fatness, or insomnia. Death, too, is one of the consequences of ageing. While ageing goes on like an engine driver putting on the brakes, death, when the engine actually stops, can occur at any time.

The causes of death can give an idea of the kinds of diseases to which a group of ageing people in a particular society are prone to. In Western countries the causes of death in the very old people (70-80) are primarily diseases of the arteries and the heart, followed by chest infections and cancer. This indicates that the circulatory system is the 'Achilles heel' of Western man, and we will be paying special attention to it in the following pages.

At younger ages (60-70) the causes of death are more related to specific diseases rather than general deterioration, thus cancer is the major killer, followed by diseases of the blood system, lung infections, and diseases of the digestive system. Bluntly put, it takes a stronger blow to fell a healthier tree – the younger you are, the nastier the disease must be to kill you, while the older you are, the more vulnerable you become to milder and milder forms of degeneration, until at very old ages it often becomes impossible to tell of which disease a person will die. This is the state that we aspire to. A long life without a nasty ending.

An Aged Body

There is no part of the body that is not affected by ageing. When we see dry wrinkled skin, it means that the invisible and essential molecules of the skin are gradually losing elasticity. We notice loss of memory, or slower reactions, but we do not see that every day up to ten thousand of the cells of the brain are lost, the minute blood-vessels supplying oxygen to these cells become blocked and ineffective. We notice that bones are broken more easily. A strange chaos is causing this inside the body, since the calcium is no longer properly contained within the bones, but leaks out and deposits itself in the soft parts of the body, hardening vessels which should be soft, softening bones which should be hard. The spine becomes compressed, changing the stature. Reduced energy is a universal result of ageing, due to changes in the metabolism, the brain and the heart.

All these changes interact with each other. For example, a malfunctioning heart will affect the water-works, and poor kidney function will affect metabolism and changed metabolism will affect everything else and so it goes on. Like a car, each part has been designed for a certain period of usefulness. The gearbox may tend to go first in one model, the chassis in another, but mostly, it is the case that in the end everything seems to fail together; to the delight of scrap yards and the motor industry alike. Our potential lifespan is fixed within narrow limits. We have built-in obsolescence.

The Choked Channels

Cazalis, the medical writer asserted, at the turn of the century, that a man was as old as his arteries. As more and more diseases are cured in our industrial civilization we are left with the most insoluble problem of all: our blood vessels.

As we get older, the walls of the vessels become tougher and tighter. Blood pressure rises as the resistance increases. In addition, small patches appear inside our blood vessels. These form a focus for the laying down of fatty deposits and, as more fat is laid down, they become hard calcified patches which block the blood vessels. They can also precipitate a blood clot inside the vessels since the clotting mechanism mistakes these patches for wounds, and this 'thrombosis', as it is called, can produce a fatal blockage or bleeding.

The two most vulnerable organs in our body are the heart and the brain. Both desperately need every last drop of oxygen-carrying blood to work with their usual high efficiency. The thirsty heart muscle, in its marathon pumping, is usually the first to be affected by blocked vessels. A small part of the heart muscle is starved of oxygen and dies: this is a heart attack. A blood-vessel of the heart is blocked by a clot: this is a coronary thrombosis. When the brain is suddenly affected by a blocked or burst vessel some brain tissue dies: this is a stroke. These are without a doubt the major causes of death in our civilization. Why do they occur? What can be done about them?

In the face of the degeneration of the blood-vessels, medicine is a helpless bystander. Cardiovascular problems are not cured, but 'managed' as the euphemism goes. It is possible to clear a clot, but not to repair the damaged heart, nor are there drugs to remove fibrous, calcified or fatty material piled up inside the arteries. How many doctors have dreamt of some medicinal agent which would scrub the inside of the arteries and leave them fresh and clear like a child's? It is, alas, a daydream. Only dietary practices can reverse the changes to a certain extent.

On the other hand, it is possible to attack it at the source, if we know how it occurs. In the past when the emotions were thought to be located in the heart, heart disease was imagined to be the result of rage and grief: 'my life is at the mercy of any fool who shall put me in a passion' wrote John Hunter, an eighteenth-century surgeon. More recently diet was thought to be the bugbear. Biochemists discovered that a high cholesterol content in the diet was linked with heart disease. This was confirmed by feeding laboratory animals on controlled diets rich in cholesterol. They did indeed suffer more frequently from circulatory disorders. The impact of these discoveries was considerable. Half a nation turned away from butter and cream which is full of cholesterol, to vegetable margarine which is not. Not so many gave up meat. But it is not so simple. Eskimos who eat seal-fat would, according to the cholesterol theory, all be dead by middle age, as would the Masai tribesmen with their milk and blood diet. Cholesterol is made by the body, and the high level could be due to manufacture rather than ingestion.

Today, authorities feel that the most insidious, far-reaching problem is the failure to deal with stress. Excess salt, or animal fats in the diet only aggravate the situation. Young pilots in the Korean and Vietnam wars were found to have an astonishing degree of arteriosclerosis. Heart disease was associated more with overwrought, anxious or aggressive people, harkening back to the 'killing-rage' theory of the eighteenth century. Our way of life is engraved on the inside of our blood-vessels, in a morse code of fatty dots and dashes.

Cancer: a Rogue Elephant

Cancer too is an unpleasant result of ageing in the modern world. One in five hospital deaths in the United States is the result of cancer. It is rare enough in primitive rural societies to be regarded as the vengeance of a particularly nasty spirit, or the consequence of especially poor morality in some previous incarnation.

We know that cancer begins with a cell or tissue that is not particularly abnormal, just undisciplined. It grows without reference to the controls exerted by the body and eventually becomes a parasite. In this case, a cancer tissue arises out of the varied activity of normal tissue like a rampaging rogue elephant within a herd of peaceful elephants. The rogue elephant is still elephant, the cancer tissue still our living material. We all have potential cancer nascent within us. The chances of activation depend on a multitude of factors including exposure to harmful chemicals, to radiation, to asbestos, to cigarette smoke, to certain types of diet, to poisonous waste products in our own body which we do not properly remove. It is thought that most of the cancers today are caused by environmental chemicals and pollutants. These build up over a lifetime and the likelihood of contracting cancer increases rapidly as one gets older.

We are not powerless to control this runaway beast, for natural resistance is tirelessly sifting the cells of the body and destroying damaged or deviant cancer cells. Thus the strength of our natural resistance is vital in preserving us from cancer as from any other disease. Psychological factors, particularly melancholia and maladaption to life, influence the likelihood of cancer. Galen, who mentioned in 540 B.C. that'melancholy women were more likely to incur cancer than sanguine women', is supported by modern research. We swim through a sea of cancer-causing agents all our lives and our resistance must be tuned to perfection to avoid this disease, as the others, on the way to old age.

3
THE QUEST FOR LONGEVITY

A poor archer draws his bow, aims, and shoots with just enough power to ensure that the arrow reaches the target, and he misses. A skilful archer tests the wind, the temperature, the atmosphere, before aiming and shoots with maximum power. He hits the target because he takes into account all the various factors which might alter the course of the arrow in its flight, especially towards the end.

We begin life, like the arrow leaving the bow, with an impetus for survival. We rise up through youth, reach our peak at adulthood and descend in old age to our lifespan target. If we skilfully manipulate our flight and descent we can reach more distant targets and we can ensure a smoother journey. Whatever guidance we give to the arrow of our lifespan must be put into practice as early as possible. The great physician Avicenna, born exactly a thousand years ago, understood this well:

> Every person has his own term of life . . . . the art of
> maintaining health consists in guiding the body to its
> natural span.

The Vales of the Blessed

From time to time reports appear of the existence of communities in which some individuals live for a remarkably long time. Usually such communities live in isolated and secluded valleys within mountain regions. In the Hunza valley of North Pakistan, a Switzerland in the foothills of the Himalayas, there are many such people, while the Andean village of Vilcabamba, Ecuador, boasted 9 individuals above 100, and 1 of 123 in a community of 819. In this case, there was evidence in the form of baptismal certificates to support the claims of the people themselves. We know the exaggerative tendencies of the human mind, and experts have always wrestled with the problem that old people tend to falsify their ages, either because they genuinely do not know, or because they desire the sense of achievement of reaching a grander old age.

The failure of experts to be careful has lead to the perpetration of a monumental fraud. It has been internationally accepted that there are extremely old people living in the Republic of Georgia, in the Caucasus mountains of the USSR. The Russians even issued a postage stamp of one such Georgian in 1956 when he was 148. He reached the purported age of 168. There were reported to be 8,890 centenarians in the area, 500 of whom were between 120 and 170. A centenarian dance troupe of fifty dancers was formed to dance in theatres from Moscow to Minsk. Thousands of physiological tests were carried out which showed them to be typical of the healthy elderly. However, quite recently Dr Zhores Medvedev, a Russian gerontologist demonstrated by means of a brilliant piece of scientific detective work that the individuals had falsified their ages as was the custom in the region. For example, he showed that life expectancy in Georgia is no more than anywhere else in the USSR and it may even be less, and while the life expectancy increased in recent years the number of centenarians actually went down. Proper statistics killed the centenarians!

Despite this amusing hocus-pocus we can accept that it is possible that in certain communities there are extremely long-lived people. They are mostly isolated and rural, poor but healthy, engaged in agriculture and living frugally. They usually live high up in mountainous regions which seem to be invigorating, clean and detached from both the diseases and the disruptions of people living nearer sea level. There is no consistency among the herbs, foods and folk practices which these people use. In fact they usually place no more emphasis on health practices than any other group of simple people. The centenarians from the Ecuador, smoke from 20 to 60 home rolled cigarettes a day! It is probable that their long life is the result of constitution, isolation, and their simple agricultural daily life.

Prolonging Life

There have been two opposing streams of thought about the wisdom of prolonging life. One holds that we should not meddle with our God-given lifespan, as Sophocles states scornfully:

Who craves excess of days
Scorning the common span
Of life, I judge that man
a giddy fellow who walks in folly's ways.

In the epic of Gilgamesh, a story traced back to the Sumerians of 3000 B.C., Gilgamesh who seeks to escape death is told: 'When the Gods created mankind they allotted death to mankind, but life they retained in their keeping'. The Epicurean philosophers made a virtue of necessity and stated that one could not, by living any longer, achieve much more than is possible in the present lifetime, and since death is waiting for us in the end anyway, it would be better to concentrate on living fully than postponing death. The Roman Stoics and the Old Testament tradition both held that death is a necessity which must be accepted not fought, while the New Testament saw it only as a precondition for resurrection.

Yet this position, based on humility under God's rule, is balanced by its exact opposite in China. Taoism, which does not teach submission to a powerful deity, developed methods of obtaining immortality as one of its essential features. The attainment of long life was a preoccupation of everyone from Taoist priests to laymen, scholars to Emperors, and this great undertaking was part of the stimulus to the early growth of science and medicine in China and has had reverberations through the ages until today. Taoist devotion to immortality is important to us for two reasons. The techniques may be of considerable value to our goal of a healthy old age, if we can understand and adapt them. Secondly, the Taoist longevity tradition has brought us many interesting remedies.

Taoism

The *Tao Te Ching* which propounds the metaphysical basis of
Taoism is one of the most subtle books known, with an equally
mysterious author, Lao Tzu. It was written around 300 B.C. In
this and other books, is poetically unfolded the existence of
the Tao, which is the underlying constant essence or character
of Nature:

> Nature does not have to insist,
> can blow for only half a morning. . .
> If nature does not have to insist
> Why should man?

The work of man is to merge with this flow, not through the
learning of names and categories, but through insight, and
quiet ecstasy.

Taoism taught a way of acting in life described by the well
known phrase *wu wei* or harmonious effortless action, which
conserved resources and increased rather than wasted energy.
This quietism brought the reward of long life which could be
increased by tapping the unlimited power of the Tao.

> Breath for men to draw from as they will
> And the more they take of it, the more remains.

Taoists held that vitality was used up in struggle and effort, but
the wise man conserved his vitality through skilful and easy
action, just as an experienced craftsman can extend the life of
his tools by using them properly. He who tapped the Tao was
regarded as free from harm and disease and eventually
became a *hsien* or immortal saint-like being. The *hsien* are the
gnarled old men, full of impish and youthful vitality, seen in
many Chinese pictures.

Taoist practices held that although the final goal was
immortality, the secret of the way took so long to find that
some initial lifespan prolongation was necessary in order to
have the time to attempt the greater task. Most Taoists were
satisfied to work for this initial lifespan prolongation and leave
the alchemical search for immortality to the sages, alchemists
and priests. For the fascinating story of the alchemical
preparation of the elixir, the reader is referred to the bibli-
ography.

The process of attaining super longevity was termed

'initiating the embryo' since it attempted to quieten body processes until it became possible to obtain food without eating, like the foetus in the womb. It is interesting that a 'return to the womb' practice appears in other traditional longevity cures, for example, the Rasaaynen therapy for longevity, which is part of the Ayurvedic Indian traditional medicine system. This system included shutting the subject within a small, sealed hut of exactly prescribed dimensions for several months, in addition to the consumption of a variety of vegetable and mineral medicines. Nehru, the famous Indian head of state, was believed to have undergone Rasaaynen therapy.

The longevity practices developed by the Taoists became the teaching of an established priesthood. They have been diligently carried out by adherents ever since. So developed did this system of practices become that it has never been bettered to this day. Writers and thinkers on longevity have, as we shall see, recommended this or that method of attaining a healthy old age, but the Taoists included and predated them all.

The Life Breath

Air has always been synonymous with life or spirit. The Greek word *psyche* originally meant breath and then came to mean spirit. The Taoists, like the Buddhists and Tantricists knew the breath to be the bridge between man and the macrocosm. The world breathed and man could gain access to this breath by modulating his own inspiration and expiration. The life giving aspect of breath was thought to be not so much in the air or oxygen, but in an energy that can be obtained from outside the body, with sufficient practice, called *chi* in the Chinese system equivalent to *prana* in the Yogic system.

The first step in Taoist breath control was breath retention, to be practiced after certain preparatory rituals. The breath was held for longer and longer times by arduous training, and serious benefit to health only became possible when the breath could be held for a time equivalent to a hundred and twenty respirations. Some adepts believed that breath holding for a time equivalent to a thousand respirations was necessary. We can also note the importance of breath holding in Yogic breathing (termed *Kumbhaka:* the crocodile), reaching a level of competence in which the Yogi can be buried alive for days before emerging unharmed.

The next stage in the Taoist practice was to direct the preserved breath, by mental concentration and visualization, to flow to various parts of the body, in particular the glands at the base of the spine, which we may regard as the glands making sexual secretions. The mixture of breath and fluid then travelled up the spine where it produced an explosively restorative effect. After this it was passed back to the throat and swallowed with saliva in its transformed state in a process termed 'nourishment by the breath'. This practice is again surprisingly similar to Tantric methods whereby certain breathing and postures awaken a kind of sexual secretion seen as a snake *(Kundalini)* which travels up the spine and, joining with elements in the brain, produces complete bliss, super longevity and miraculous powers.

Scientifically there is no reason why, given sufficient practice, breath retention could not be extended for very long periods. It would be accompanied by gradual adaptation to a more efficient retrieval and a reduced demand for oxygen, in other words a quietening of the entire metabolism into a state akin to hibernation. These adaptations though difficult to attain would tend to produce a longer life, for lung capacity and oxygen transport is one of the limiting factors in our lifespan, and metabolic rate is also connected to longevity. Holding of breath would expand the blood vessels in the brain and the body tissues and keep them in better condition. The *Kundalini* practice is so mysterious that few have attempted to impose on it crude medical speculation.

The Food Problem

The most famous of long-lived Englishmen was Thomas Parr, known as Old Parr, who is widely reported to have lived to 152. Contemporary records are in no doubt that he lived long because of his simple regular life and his minimal vegetarian diet:

> Good wholesome labour was his exercise,
> Down with the lamb, and with the lark would rise;
> In mire and toiling sweat he spent the day,

And to his team he whistled time away:
The cock his night-clock, and till day was done,
His watch and chief sun-dial was the sun.
He was of old Pythagoras' opinion,
That new cheese was most wholesome with an onion;
Coarse meslin bread, and for his daily swig,
Milk, butter-milk, and water, whey and whig;
Sometimes metheglin, and, by fortune happy,
He sometimes sipped a cup of ale most nappy,
Cyder, or perry, when he did repair
To a Whitson-ale, wake, wedding, or a fair,
Or when in Christmas-time he was a guest
At his good landlord's house among the rest;
Else he had little leisure time to waste,
Or at the ale-house, buff-cup ale to taste;
His physic was good butter, which the soil
Of Salop yields, more sweet than Candy oil;
And garlic he esteemed above the rate
Of Venice treacle, or best mithridate
He entertained no gout, no ache he felt,
The air was good and temperate where he dwelt;
Thus living within bounds of nature's laws,
Of his long lasting life may be some cause.

Indeed his death was a touching statement of this principle. When he was invited to visit King Charles I to be honoured on the occasion of his 150th birthday he was encouraged to eat meat and delicacies and after a life of simple vegetarian foods the extravagance in his honour killed him.

Thomas Parr and the Hunza valley centenarians had one specific feature in common: temperance. Before we say that we have heard it all before as in the hypocritical preachings of the Victorian age, let us hasten to add that temperance means removing excesses, which implies cutting down waste. Waste is poisonous, whether on the planet or inside the body. Restriction of the intake of food is the most consistent advice offered on prolonging life by almost every expert on the question. The Chinese teach us always to leave the table with a little bit of hunger remaining, a longevity maxim continually repeated by Gandhi. The Taoists advised strict principles of austerity in the diet so as to avoid contamination by the formation of 'impure' excrements. One meal was taken each day, and this contained only roots, berries, fruits and nuts.

The Taoists were strictly against grains. Tao Tsang wrote:

> The five cereals are the scissors which cut down life,
> they destroy the vital organs, they shorten the lifespan.

All the great writers on medicine from Aristotle to Avicenna taught that diet restriction brought health. The Renaissance writer, Luigi Cornaro, for example, suffered a serious disease at 40, through overindulgence, which induced him to severely cut down his food intake. He recovered his health and was not affected by any further ailment until the age of 75 when he fell ill, which, he maintained, was solely because for once he listened to the blandishment of his gluttonous friends and ate heartily. He cured himself by frugality, living to 91 and losing no opportunity to tell the world all about it: 'I feel when I leave the table I must sing'.

Food and Ageing: Medical Evidence

Medical research has now confirmed the value of these dietary practices in two areas. Firstly, that excess food can encourage various diseases of advanced age, and secondly, that minimal diets can almost double the lifespan of experimental animals. It is somewhat incredible that despite the vast resources of the medical world and the libraries full of medical books on curing diseases by every kind of surgery and medicament, the only positive medical statements about preventing diseases of old age and attaining long life are exactly identical to the intuitive observations of Thomas Parr, Cornaro and others, which cost not a penny in research funds and were worked out without an army of statisticians and gerontologists.

The story of the over-consumption of animal foods is too well known to bear repetition and although, as we have seen, the state of our blood-vessels owes more to our general level of stress than to this or that item of diet alone, the advice against animal fats is sound. There are unfortunately few medical studies on the medical effects of vegetarianism but any doctor can tell you that vegetarians have a lower blood pressure than non-vegetarians. Meat eating and spicy foods have been associated with cancer of the intestines or bowels. Moreover, there is a theory propounded by several well known experts that rich food, without fibrous material (e.g. white bread rather than brown, and a lack of vegetables) may tend to produce cancer, for it passes so slowly through the intestine that it putrefies on the way and forms poisonous and cancer-causing waste products. It is also worth remembering that the simpler the food the less chance for contamination by pollutants and poisons which, we now know, are a major cause of cancers of various kinds.

In 1939 Dr McKay, originally working on behalf of life insurance, published the results of a long study of food consumption and lifespan in the laboratory rat. He found something extraordinary which has intrigued everyone concerned with ageing and nutrition. When his animals were given a diet deficient in calories during the first part of their lives, they grew more slowly and they lived to very much greater ages. They seemed to be more alert and healthy and contracted fewer chronic diseases, especially cancer. If diet was poor only late in life there were improvements in lifespan but not nearly as great as the long term treatment. As a recent article by Dr Ross stated:

> Chronic underfeeding of a complete diet is the only means known for increasing the length of life of laboratory animals beyond the limits characteristic of their species. At the other extreme, chronic overfeeding or other dietary excesses or imbalances curtails lifespan.

Ross found that when laboratory rodents were allowed to select their own diets from a range of possible diets both rich and poor, the animals that ate less in early life lived much longer. The longest-lived rats were the ones that consumed a diet with sufficient protein but low carbohydrate and fat early in life (i.e. before maturity) and very little protein later in life.

The same considerations are likely to apply to man. We know that very long-lived people such as the Hunza valley centenarians eat very little, indeed their diet has been calculated to contain on average 1,200 calories a day which is half that recommended by medical authorities. The dangers of overeating after maturity are also evident because of diseases like diabetes and atherosclerosis and because a high protein diet is known to be more likely to harm the kidneys and may cause rheumatic problems. There are many reports and anecdotes on recovery from diseases through near starvation. For example, in one concentration camp in the last war during a typhus outbreak, 100 per cent of the well-fed German guards were affected by the disease but only 30 per cent of the starving Russian inmates. Undernourished (but not completely starved) children were found to be much more resistant to serious virus infections such as polio and hepatitis during a recent drought in Africa. There seems to be strong confirmation of the suggestion by Cornaro that:

> Nature being desirous to preserve man as long as possible teaches what role to follow in time of illness for she immediately deprives the sick of their appetite in order that they may eat but little, for with little, Nature is content.

Gymnastic Techniques

The Taoists were well aware that respiratory longevity practices could only be effectively carried out in a healthy body. Systems of exercises were therefore developed to lay the foundation for other practices as well as to promote longevity in their own right. The Taoist techniques are again not dissimilar to the Yoga asanas or positional exercises. They have both produced Western offshoots, for the Taoist techniques influenced the Western medical gymnastics of today, through the founder of the Swedish system of medical gymnastics, Dr Henrik Ling, while the Hatha Yoga asanas of Patanjali generated the 'T.V. Yoga' of today. The Taoists felt that exercise cleared obstructions or blockages to the proper flow of the breath of life force around the body, much as the modern doctor will confirm that exercise aids the circulation and prevents blockages of the arteries. Tai Ch'i is a present day Chinese exercise system, now becoming popular in the West which illustrates the principles of the techniques, which can be described by 'wu wei' – effortless action. The exercises require great strength and control, but they must be achieved with maximum economy and grace. The classic Taoist postures are carried out squatting on the floor, and consist of stretching and twisting, bending forwards and backwards, neck rotation and isometric contractions of the muscles. They are, like Yoga, accompanied by controlled breathing which has the purpose of aiding balance and concentration as well as improving the lungs and circulation. The well known Buddha statues of the

Far East often show him sitting with hands pushed high in the air, palms to heaven, in a typical Taoist exercise position.

Yoga is much more sophisticated with thousands of postures of graded severity, each with specific effects on different body systems. The effect of Yoga on the circulation is truly magnificent, and medicine has hardly scratched the surface in examining the benefits attributable to Yoga postures or more correctly, the way of life of a Hatha Yogi, the postures being only one part of the path. The inverse postures, that is the head stand or shoulder stand are of particular importance for longevity, for they increase the blood circulation in the brain and maintain flexibility of its blood-vessels. There is an additional effect on the hormone systems which we have seen are critically important for a healthy old age. The brain contains the hypothalamus and pituitary, two small glands which control the response of most of the other hormone-producing glands of the body. The inverse Yoga postures are thought to improve the function of these vital glands and thereby maintain the resistance and vitality of the body and extend the lifespan. Other Yoga postures, the twists, stomach contractions and so on are also thought to stimulate the secretions of various glands to maintain their adequate function for longer than normal. This particularly includes the sexual glands, Yoga being a specific regimen for increasing sexual vitality and energy. A recent study at Benaras Hindu University recorded profound improvements in the level of the sexual and stress protecting hormones in middle aged volunteers after a course of Yoga lasting only six months. The prestigious medical publication, *The Lancet*, reported that the Yoga method of inducing relaxation was effective in reducing blood pressure in patients with circulatory problems.

There is, of course, much medical research on the health benefits to be gained by ordinary exercise. Maintaining muscular strength and efficiency by continued exercise keeps the heart muscles and arteries in trim. Cardiologists have repeatedly warned that lack of exercise is one of the main causative factors in the premature degeneration of the blood system and the heart. 'If you want to know how flabby your brain is, feel your leg muscles'. Other studies report that hormones such as insulin which manage the energy supply of the body, become more responsive and accurate after exercise training. In other words they can adjust the flow of food, converting it more completely into energy. Hormone failure is one cause of the circulation of fats around the body which aggravates circulatory problems. Exercise has profound effects on breath capacity, reducing bronchitic problems in old age. Exercise, once begun, can be kept up steadily. Borotra was world tennis champion at fifty-six, and there are the well-known elderly people who break the ice on the Serpentine in London for their swim. Exercise should be steady. Champion athletes sometimes overdo it and their heart suffers from the stress of overexhaustion. Old people should avoid violent exercises for the same reason. The best kind of exercise is occupational, such as agriculture, which is stress-free, rhythmic and coordinated, ensuring balance and activity in muscles, nerves and breath. It is no accident that all the famous centenarian peoples are engaged in small scale agriculture.

The 'Essence'

In 1889 Professor Charles Brown-Sequard announced to the doctors of Paris that he felt thirty years younger as a result of injecting himself with extracts made from the testicles of animals. His announcement was greeted with derision and he died a few years later. Subsequently, the male sex hormone, testosterone, was found to be made in the testicles. Testosterone therapy, the modern version of Brown-Sequards testicular extract, can increase vitality and sexual vigour and is useful in the cure of certain types of male impotence. However, the improvement is short-lived and it may not have any effect on the lifespan as a whole. The same can be said of 'H.R.T.' – Hormone Replacement Therapy, much in vogue with American women but relatively unknown in Britain. This seeks to replace the oestrogen lost when the ovary ceases to function at menopause. It is useful in preventing uncomfortable menopausal symptoms and some women say it makes them feel rejuvenated. Some gynaecologists feel that it can improve complexion and skin, strengthen the bones and help prevent coronary thrombosis, which is rare in women before menopause but does occur afterwards. There is little information on the long term effects of hormone replacement in women or men. Despite some womens' enthusiasm over the oestrogen 'happy pill', there are risks of unpleasant side effects. There is also a risk that continual use will suppress whatever levels of hormone are still made by the body with opposite effects to those intended in long term.

If the artificial use of male hormones in organic or chemical form has a doubtful effect on longevity, are there other ways of increasing and maintaining the level of activity of these hormones? It seems from ancient sources that sexual practice itself can be used to increase the lifespan, and we may conclude that in so far as these practices have a vitalizing or rejuvenating effect on the whole organism it is the hormones which are the agents. The Taoists maintained that each act of sexual intercourse which resulted in an ejaculation decreased the lifespan because the loss of the 'ching' or 'essence' which went out with the seminal fluid. This belief is a strong thread running through many cultures. It is the basis of the rule of celibacy in ascetic and monastic groups. Yet the Taoists did not like celibacy which they felt to be abnormal and unhealthy. One source records:

> If man is without woman, he becomes agitated, his spirits become fatigued, if his spirits become fatigued his longevity is decreased.

Instead they practiced sexual intercourse but without ejaculation. In this way they felt they had the best of both worlds. By this means they sought not only to conserve but to augment their 'ching'.

A similar principle is found in the well-known practice of 'shunamitism', well known because of its use to vitalize the ageing King David. A young girl, Abishag of Shunam, was brought to lie with the king in non-sexual embrace. This practice, based on the belief of some rejuvenating power in the 'breath', 'heat' or 'exhalation' of young girls, became well known in the seventeenth and eighteenth centuries. We might venture to suggest that any rejuvenation achieved was the result of undischarged arousal in the older person, leading to increased sexual hormone production.

Concluding Remarks

Naturally the preceding ideas on prolonging life should not be taken as a promise for extra decades for any elderly person who wishes to go rushing off and immediately stop breathing, starve, plunge into icy rivers or indulge in exotic Taoist sexual practice. These practices when properly applied are a life's work. When old age arrives much harm has already been done. It is clear from the diet restriction experiments as well as other kinds of evidence, that any procedure which may be suitably applied to produce longevity must be practiced through as much of the lifespan as possible. The above methods for prolongevity can be used undiluted by younger people who should obtain the necessary instruction as described in the concluding chapter. Older people need to take their changes easily. No abrupt or traumatic alterations of life habits and accustomed patterns of living will help the older person even if the new pattern which emerges is potentially more healthy.

Although much can be done by ordinary people who are not Taoist alchemists, there are limits. The main limit is constitutional. Constitution implies a set of qualities inherited from parents or ancestors. Just as height is inherited, or hair colour, so potential lifespan is inherited, although the similarity between parents and children is only a quarter of that found with height. Twins, for example, tend to live for roughly the same length of time and they age similarly – they may suffer from the same diseases, have white hair at the same age, and so on. Animal breeders are well aware of the fact that particular breeds of cattle for example will have a known lifespan and tend to suffer from certain specific diseases: their constitution is written in their pedigrees.

Constitution provides us with a potential, the maximum distance that the archer's arrow can fly. The methods we have described will allow more people to reach their potential without deteriorating prematurely. Some idea of the possibilities are given by the widely quoted projection that if the degenerative diseases of ageing are conquered, it will add another fifteen years to our average life expectancy. It would make many of us centenarians.

4
PLANT REMEDIES FOR THE ELDERLY IN EAST AND WEST

The use of herbs in Chinese medicine is an ancient tradition harking back to the verbal teaching of the legendary founder of agriculture and herbal medicine, the Emperor Shen Nung who, some say, lived in 3000 B.C. The tradition was systematized in a classic work on herbal medicine, the *Pen-ts'ao Kangmu,* compiled by Li Shih-chen at the end of the sixteenth century, which included 10,000 herbal prescriptions.

The medicines were roughly divided into three groups:
1. The mild herbs which are also harmless, and used for health maintenance (kingly),
2. Somewhat stronger herbs which are relatively non-toxic (princely),
3. Powerful herbs which are at the same time potentially toxic, and which are used as curative medicine if initial mild treatments fail to prevent disease (assistant).

Most of the prescriptions in this Pharmacopoeia are used today when the materials are available.

For the elderly, many of the most useful herbs are of a mild restorative nature. They are used to increase vitality and energy, and strengthen resistance against disease. Such herbs are given for very long periods and are usually extremely expensive. They are mostly used in combination.

Ginseng is the single most useful restorative and tonic available in China and the Far East. It is a component of a multitude of remedies and preparations, especially where old

people are concerned, but in each case ginseng is not the
curative element. Thus in plant concoctions, it is used to assist
a curative agent by increasing whole-body energy, vitality and
resilience, or to give supporting strength during treatment and
convalescence. It may be combined, for example, with roasted
and skinned deer horn, a preparation called 'panty'. A typical
tonic preparation for the elderly could be:

> ginseng root
> liquorice root
> *Atractylis ovata*
> *Poria cocos*
> ginger
> jujube berries

which are boiled for extensive periods together.

What is Ginseng?

Ginseng is the root of the plant *Panax ginseng* (C.A. Meyer). It is
the romanization of the Chinese name jen-shen or 'man-
essence'. Shen is applied to many medicinal roots and has the
meaning of a crystallization of the essence of the earth in a
form beneficial to man. There are a multitude of Chinese
names for ginseng, reflecting millenia of romantic enthusiasm
for their most important medicinal plant. Interestingly, the
name also refers to the constellation of Orion which is man-
like in shape and imagined by the Chinese to have an astral
influence on the plant. Panax is the botanic name of the small
genus to which ginseng belongs, within the family of *Araliaceae*.
It was given to the genus by the great taxonomist Linnaeus
because he was aware of the usefulness of ginseng. It heralds
from the Greek *pan-akos* or all-healing.

Panax ginseng used to grow wild in China and Korea, and it
was collected with considerable ritual, solemnity and, of
course, avidity. Nowadays it is becoming rare in many areas
through overcropping. One or two wild roots are found every
year in Korea, and more in the Sikhote-Alin mountains of East
Manchuria and the Eastern Siberian seaboard. Wild ginseng
and the best quality Imperial ginseng previously grown in the
royal parks are the most prized and expensive herbs known to
man. Only recently a Chinese pharmacist in New York stated

that he would offer $10,000 for a top quality wild ginseng root. The huge specimen on display in Moscow's Achievements Exhibition has been valued at 25,000 roubles. Wild ginseng is regarded as more valuable in part because it is often very old. The Russians claim to have found roots which are hundreds of years old (judged by the wrinkles on the neck of the root), but there is no way to judge if this is true. The ginseng currently available are the cultivated roots, grown in Korea or China which are classed according to age, consistency and size. Some ginseng is specially selected and treated by scraping, steaming over a vessel on a fire of special wood, followed by drying. This gives it a red, glassy appearance. A good red ginseng root, though cultivated, is customarily regarded as a better quality than the white roots. The Chinese prepare a sugared ginseng from older roots which are pricked and bathed repeatedly in a sugar solution. There is also an American species *Panax quinquefolium*, and various types of *Panax pseudoginseng*. However, the latter are not strictly comparable as they are used in the Far East for different purposes. For example, *Panax pseudoginseng var. japonicus* is used to disperse extravasated blood, in swellings, bruises and internal haemorrhage.

Ginseng is surrounded by a great web of mystery, superstition, fancy and greed. It is similar in this regard to the mandrake root, a completely unrelated plant with which it is often confused. The extravagance with which herbalists and patients make claims for ginseng, as well as other herbs, is astonishing but understandable, considering the mystery of healing and the human capacity for enthusiasm. Yet it must not serve as an *a priori* reason either to reject or accept. Instead, these claims should be used as a basis for further investigation, particularly when almost half the world believes implicitly in them. It forces us at least to sit up and take notice.

Ginseng and the Elderly Chinese

Ginseng increases in value with the age of the root. It also increases in value with the age of the person desiring it. Some old Chinese spend their life savings on a single gnarled root or an extract. When a root is obtained, the purchaser chops it in small pieces and boils them all night over a slow fire in a special silver kettle. No ferrous metals are permitted to come into contact with the root. Before dawn the old man or woman gets up, drinks the decoction, chews the fibrous solids and returns to sleep. During the time he takes the root, which may be for a few weeks to many months depending on his pocket, he is quiet and celibate, eating as simple a diet as possible. He believes that the vitality which ginseng generates can be all too easily squandered by using up the energy in sexual activity or in stressful experiences or overindulgence.

Some old people keep ginseng in brandy for years, taking out the conditioned brandy in times of need or illness, or in company with honoured guests. It was common practice to procure some ginseng as a last minute restorative at the time of dying, so that the moribund individual would arrange his affairs, and depart to join his ancestors in good order and in prayer or meditation.

There is as much appreciation of ginseng in China today as there has been in the past years, the only difference being a wider circle of ginseng cognoscenti all over the world, and the almost total unavailability of the best Imperial and wild ginseng. Yet China and particularly Korea export huge quantities of cultivated root. Mao-tse-tsung and Chou-en-lai reportedly took it as do the hierarchy in North Vietnam. Senior Russian and Far Eastern diplomats take it, and so do the Saudi and Middle Eastern potentates. It is standard fare of ageing politicians and showbiz personalities in the U.S.A.

> Publick Fame saith that the popes of Rome, who are chosen to that office when they are very old doe make great use of this root to preserve their Radical moysture and natural Heat, that so they may the longer enjoy their Comfortable Preferments . . .

wrote William Simpson in 1680 in a letter to the Royal Society. Things have not changed since.

Traditional Claims and Uses

The claims made for ginseng in earlier oriental herbal compendia, and in reports arising from China, are extravagant indeed. They state that ginseng is nothing less than a panacea that can virtually bring life to the dead. This exaggeration has served both to entrance people with the potent image of a near magical medicine, and create a sceptical backlash against the root in the medical world of the West. In fact, the wild claims can be understood as enthusiastic metaphors, used by traditional herbalists of the time in China, and similarly by earlier herbalists in Europe. It is part of the language, particularly in the Chinese idiographic script which even describes modern drugs with exotic descriptive apellations. Tranquillizers, in Chinese script, become 'pills which bring rest to the eyes'. Another reason for the extravagant early claims is that they are based on the use of the wild ginseng root which is very much more powerful than today's cultivated root, and now unobtainable. A third reason is a misunderstanding. The Chinese state that ginseng acts on many body systems together, rather than on a single organ or a single disease entity. This statement has been misunderstood and reinterpreted by Western observers to mean some kind of panacea.

The Chinese currently use it as a general restorative to increase strength and stamina, to overcome weakness in old age and convalescence, to restore potency lost through age or trauma, to adjust blood-pressure and blood sugar, (in combination with other drugs) to reduce agitation and nervous tension as well as anaemia. It is used by the army in case of wounding, and as a prophylactic for those at risk of disease or injury. A proportion of these claims have been investigated in pharmacological laboratories, and these findings will be discussed in the next chapter.

A reasonable distillation of traditional claims reduces them down to one: that ginseng is an extremely effective restorative. The earliest statement on ginseng in the legendary pharmacopoeia of the 'Heavenly Husbandman', is still one of the best:

> It is used for repairing the five viscera (this applies to metabolic processes rather than organs - S.F.) harmonising energies, strengthening the soul, allaying fear, removing toxic substances, brightening the eyes, opening the heart, and improving thought. Continuous use will invigorate the body and prolong life.

The Chinese see ginseng as repairing the 'yang', that is increasing heat, activity and metabolic turnover in the body and particularly in the brain. The improved mental function, alertness and memory that is obtained through the use of ginseng is also an increase in *yang*.

In contrast to the exotic claims made for *Panax ginseng*, the reported traditional usage of the American species, *Panax quinquefolium*, is much more limited. The french Canadians call it *garantogin*, and use it for asthma, stomach complaints and the promotion of female fertility. The American Indians used it regularly as a medicinal plant but, as one commentator observed, 'they do not so highly esteem the Ginseng as their Tartar brethren in Asia do'. It was used in cold and cough medicines, especially by the Greeks, who mixed it with ginger and alchohol to promote sweating. In general, the traditional interest in ginseng in America was in digging it up to export it to China rather than in consuming it at home. However, in recent years there has been a large upswing in the reputation of ginseng, especially among the young in America, and *panax quinquefolium* is also being collected to extinction.

Other Araliaceous Tonic Plants

Euleutherococcus senticosus belongs to the same Araliaceous family as ginseng. It is a thorny shrub with long rhizomes, creeping under the soil. The rhizomes have been used in Chinese medicine as a kind of poor-man's ginseng. Because the plant grows wild in large quantities both in China and the USSR, it has supplanted ginseng as the prime tonic remedy. It has also flooded Western countries. 15 per cent of all 'ginseng' sold in the U.K. is in fact *Eleutherococcus senticosus* often called 'Siberian ginseng'.

Although the Chinese used *eleutherococcus* as a general tonic which they called *ciwuja*, they always thought of it as inferior to real ginseng. That is, until the supplies of real high quality ginseng became scarce. As the quality of mass cultivated ginseng dropped, the possibilities of substitutes were re-explored both at the folk level and in the institutes of traditional medicine and pharmacology. Looking into *eleutherococcus* more closely, the Russians and Chinese realized that it had one or two genuine advantages over ginseng. *Eleutherococcus* was not as stimulatory as ginseng, and therefore there was less chance of possible side-effects such as overstimulation, insomnia and agitation. These can occur when ginseng is taken by certain naturally speedy constitutional types, especially in concert with caffeinated beverages. The second advantage is that it is equally valid for men and women, while ginseng is predominantly a male 'yang' remedy, increasing male hormonal activity. However, both these advantages of *eleutherococcus* are really only relevant to younger people. For older people, the Chinese unreservedly recommend ginseng, even if of poorer quality, for its heating, restorative actions are precisely those needed by old people.

The biggest boost to *eleutherococcus* has come not from the traditional Chinese at all, but from modern Soviet Union. *Eleutherococcus* is not a traditional medicine in the Soviet folk history. However, it was investigated in the laboratory at the Institute of Biologically Active Substances in Vladivostok. This research was a part of a large programme to discover new kinds of tonic and preventive remedies, from the Araliaceous plant family. As a result of the tests to be described in the next chapter, *eleutherococcus* was elevated to being one of the prime candidates for the most suitable tonic for widespread distribution throughout the USSR. In 1962, *eleutherococcus* was authorised by the Soviet health ministry to be distributed as a tonic medicine. At present *eleutherococcus* is harvested from the forests of Eastern USSR, to supply soviet citizens with 12 million month-long courses per year. Ginseng by contrast is only grown on one or two state farms, and it is largely reserved for research purposes. Much of the *eleutherococcus* sold in the USSR is taken by middle-aged or elderly people as a restorative. It is prescribed quite widely for this purpose by soviet doctors. However, it is also used in hospitals to aid recovery and to increase patients' resistance, especially after therapeutic radiation or operations. It is used by people under physiological stress, such as explorers, cosmonauts, seamen or athletes, often under direct instruction from government agencies.

New uses are being discovered for it all the time. These usually turn on the potential for *eleutherococcus* to strengthen general health and vitality during the course of specific treatments; 80,000 car workers at the huge Togliatti automobile works on the Volga river have been given lengthy *eleutherococcus* treatments. It seems that the incidence of high blood-pressure was thereby reduced, although it is hard to firmly establish a causal connection. *Eleutherococcus* like ginseng, is given as a supplementary remedy during the treatment of high blood-pressure and other cardiovascular diseases in clinics in the USSR. It appears to aid in the stabilization of blood-pressure in an indirect manner – by improving control over internal body states. Soviet studies highlighted the fact that only in chronic and debilitating disease can *eleutherococcus* be expected to be of real benefit, for in these, recovery of the patient does depend on general vitality, energy and resistance. For example, trials at the Neurology Institute of the USSR Academy of Sciences have shown improved recovery in long-term patients suffering from debility and nervous complications of several diseases. Similar trials were reported at the Pulmonary Institute in the case of chronic bronchical diseases, and the Khabarovsk Medical Institute in the case of chronic tuberculosis.

Russian research has uncovered some similar properties in other plants of the same family, though none have come out of the tests with such flying colours as their prize *eleutherococcus*. *Aralia tetrapanax, Aralia cordata,* and *Aralia manshurica* have tonic properties, while *Acanthopanax sessiliflorum* is extremely close to *Eleutherococcus senticosus* both botanically and chemically. It is sometimes used as a substitute for *eleutherococcus* in European preparations of 'siberian ginseng', although its effects are wilder and its research pedigree is minimal. While these plants have been shown to be tonic or stimulatory in Soviet laboratory trials, their use in folk medicine is unknown and their special relevance to the elderly is uncertain.

Deer Horn and Other Oriental Restoratives

'Panty' is the name of the young horns of the noble spotted deer *(Cervus dyborskii)* which used to live in the Ussuri region of the Soviet Far East and China. Nowadays they are only available on Government farms in the Vladivostok area where the horns are used for research. Both the Chinese and the Russians place great value on the horns from this species, although one or other related deer species is mostly used since the correct species is often unavailable. The Chinese stated that the very young deer horns were a powerful rejuvenating tonic, second only to ginseng root in potency. It is used to combat fatigue, impotence, loss of memory and appetite and degenerative conditions of old age. In both Russia and China an alcoholic extract of the horns is now made on a large scale.

Research has found it to contain *pantocrine*, as the active principle.

The borderline between prescriptions for longevity and those for bolstering energy sources within the body is virtually non-existent. All longevity preparations include heating and energy producing (tonifying) herbs such as *Cornus officinalis* (cornelian cherry) or *Aloe chinsnsis* (a type of aloe). *Acorus calamus* (sweet flag) is used as a restorative in Chinese medicine as it is in the West. Other herbs used in traditional preparations stimulate the hormone-producing glands, such as the famous Tan-shen *(Salvia miltiorrhiza*, a type of sage) or *Paenia suffructicosa* (a variety of peony). Jujube berries, ginger, camphor, ground tortoiseshell, the stomach contents of the musk ox, and the consumption of large quantities of sesame are all important components of longevity prescriptions.

A well known tonic remedy in China is the red berries of *Schizandra chinensis*, known in the Eastern USSR as 'limonka' or 'Korean red berries'. These berries contain *schizandrin*, a complex chemical which Chinese scientists have recently shown to be an effective brain tonic. Hunters and travellers usually take these berries as their sole food and have recorded how alert it keeps them. It is widely used as a tonic for the elderly in China.

Oriental Elixirs

There have also been many attempts to find fabled elixirs of life in China. As Palos points out, many thought that *Eoptis teeta* was the one, others that it was *Daphne genkwa*. Even more people, both Chinese and foreign observers have assumed it to be ginseng. New candidates occasionally come to light. One venerable Chinese herbalist was Professor Li Chung Yun, who, according to official Chinese records, died in 1933 aged 256 years. He attributed his longevity to the combined use of ginseng and a herb called *fo-ti-teng* which is *Hydrocotyle asiatica minor* (Asiatic pennywort) according to Richard Lucas. This plant is, interestingly, also used in Indian medicine as a restorative and brain tonic. However there is a minority opinion that *fo-ti-teng* is *Polygonum multiflori*, the fleece flower plant, which is a classical Chinese medicine. In any event one can buy *Hydrocotyle asiatica* as *fo-ti-teng* in health shops in the

U.K. There have been few experimental studies on it apart from the demonstration that it reduces blood-pressure. There is a Chinese divine mushroom of immortality that has become enshrined in Chinese culture and represented endlessly on paintings, jade carvings, furniture, and carpets. It is called *ling chih* and is a classical symbol of happy destiny, good health and longevity. From the ample pictorial representations it has been suggested that *ling chih* is a woody fungus called *Ganoderma lucidum.* It is stunningly beautiful, with a hard and shiny top. Under certain circumstances the growth pattern changes to produce a strange deer-antler shape instead of the more usual spindly mushroom form. This is exactly the kind of transformation that makes myths out of mushrooms.

The Taoist alchemical tradition generated families of mineral remedies which were supposed to be rejuvenatory. These consisted of compounds of mercury, such as cinnabar, of antimony, gold, calomel and unknown mixtures. While such minerals are used today, their application is restricted to the treatment of serious diseases. The use of such minerals in search of eternal youth may have been successful with the original alchemists when applied with their transcendental knowledge. However, many since then have died in the attempt, for these minerals are toxic. Li Shih-chen, who compiled the main classical pharmacopoeia of Chinese herbal medicine, ridiculed these efforts, ascribing them to ignorant people who aped the alchemists.

Restorative Remedies from Other Areas

In Indian traditional medicine there are a variety of herbal remedies and practices which are used for maximizing the lifespan. This 'Rasaaynen therapy' is an entire section of the vast traditional medical treatises, dealing with the attainment of a healthy old age. It describes remedies and procedures which vary according to the age of the person, the season, and so on. Thus in the 60-70 age group, the dominant kind of remedy should be 'vajikara' remedies, for example *Mucuna prurieus.* Different plants must be taken for different constitutions and at different times of the year within this general group. At age 20-30, further back down the lifespan, another group of remedies is appropriate, including *Phyllanthus emblica.*

It is interesting that classical drugs used in Rasaaynen therapy include those also used in Chinese medicine for longevity purposes. *Hydrocotyle asiatica* appears in ageing recipes, as does liquorice, an important traditional medicine the world over. One of the most famous of Indian remedies is *Brahmi (Bacopa monniera)*. This plant contains active principles which are saponins and extremely close in structure to some of the ginseng saponins.

Although there is very little scientific work on Rasaaynen therapy, one paper has appeared reporting a study in which volunteers aged between 60 and 70 were given Rasaynen therapy every day for three months. A number of physiological parameters were improved including blood composition, liver activity, breath volume, and cardiovascular function. Of particular importance is the finding that considerably more testosterone, the male sex hormone, was made by the testicular tissues of the volunteers after the therapy.

Every traditional society has its stock of remedies to be taken during the lifespan so as to prolong life. The remedies are normally used for short-term as well as long-term functions with a tonic and energizing effect in the short term. A typical remedy of this kind is *kava-kava*, which is the root of the *Piper methysticum*, a plant found in the South Seas Islands. It is used as a general tonic and relaxant, at the same time as a potential longevity preparation. Recently a resin extracted from this plant, named kawain, has been found to clear up pigmented age-deposits which clutter up aged cells and tissues.

Western Herbal Remedies

There are a host of herbal preparations available in the West which are derived from traditional sources. They are of varying effectiveness, but in general, the restorative preparations are less efficacious than their Eastern counterparts. This is because the power and variety of medicinal plants grown in China is unexcelled, as is the sophistication of the herbal wisdom. The European ecology simply cannot produce the rich crop of medicinal plants grown in the Orient. For example, there is nothing in the West to equal ginseng root for gerontological use, and we will show why in the next chapter.

Herbs are usually prepared in the form of decoctions or

teas. Kourenoff reports one Ukranian remedy for old age
debility:

> Grind one pound of garlic, add it to a jar with the juice of 24
> lemons and leave covered for 24 days. After which take one
> teaspoon at night.

Garlic is also used in a similar Siberian remedy: 6 oz of garlic
and ½ lb of onions are gound finely, to which is added 2
tablespoonsful of cider vinegar. This is left standing in a warm
place for 24 hours, after which it is mixed with ½ lb of clear
heated honey and left for 7 days in a warm place; 4 tea-
spoonsful are taken per day. This medicine is to be taken
continuously and is said to have a cumulative effect, and be
helpful to those severely handicapped by debility, fatigue and
heart problems in old age. A large spoonful of ground horse-
radish five times a day followed by water is also recommended
against fatigue in advanced age in Russia. The common
potato, finely ground and raw, is a common remedy for the
elderly in Eastern Europe, and is said to protect against
atherosclerosis.

Many classic plant remedies have a mild but generally
beneficial effect, providing they are given 'room' to work,
without, for example, competition from heavy diets which are
anyway contrary to the goal of health in old age. One such tea
is Chamomile *(Anthemis nobilis)*, known from Egyptian times
and used as a mild sedative and aid to digestion and the
passage of food through the intestine.

A competent digestion is critical in the attempt to arrive at
old age in good condition. Looking at records of our traditional
system it may seem, at first sight, to have an almost obsessive
devotion and attention to affairs of the intestines. Herbs are
taken to aid appetite, reduce it, to increase digestion, remove
gas, to alter the motions, prevent colic and so on, and the sense
behind this preoccupation is often obscure. Fortunately, there
has been some research into the results of chronically poor
digestion. Besides causing unpleasant infections of the lower
intestines such as colitis and diverticulitis, poorly digested
food produces poisons, which cause secondary symptoms of
tiredness and ill-health throughout the body. Dr Dennis
Burkitt, the eminent British cancer epidemiologist, has recently
strongly supported the view that a slow passage of food

through the intestines leads to the formation of poisons which can cause cancer.

Remedies with a special relevance to the aged are often found to have hormonal or brain tonic effects, just as in Oriental medicine. Herbs such as alfalfa, liquorice, clover, block cohosh, or burdock have hormonal type effects and may be taken to regulate metabolism. Wormwood and other plants from the Artemesia family are regarded as brain tonics and useful for debility and poor vitality. Other tonic plants include motherwort, damiana, golden rod, peppermint, serpentaria and yarrow. Sage is an important general herb for improving strength, metabolism and general health, and is used widely for this purpose, especially in the Middle East.

A plant that used to be used adjustively and as a general tonic was *Smilax sarsaparilla*. It was taken especially in Victorian times as a health drink called 'sarsaparilla', recommended especially for those getting on in years. It has been found to contain compounds quite similar to those in the ginseng root. Indeed American sarsaparilla is made from a different plant, the spikenard, *Aralia racemosa*, which is related botanically to the ginseng group of plants. The spikenards are taken by the elderly as restoratives in traditional American folk medicine, and are used by the American Indians against exhaustion and debility.

A Belgian preparation (Waldcraft) which also contains ginseng is an example of a mixture of mild herbs, suitable for maintaining health in later life, and is formulated according to the European herbal tradition:

> Ginseng root *(Panax ginseng)*
> Balm leaves *(Melissa officinalis)**
> Hops flowers *(Humulus Lupulus)*
> Rue *(Ruta graveolens)*
> Rosemary *(Rosmarinus officinalis)*
> Dill *(Peucedanum graveolus)*
> Melitot *(Melitotus officinalis)*
> Red Clover *(Trifolium pratense)*
> Sweet Marjoram *(Origanum marjorana)*
> Chamomile flowers *(Anthemis nobilis)*
> Calamus rhizome *(Acorus calamus)*
> Gentian root *(Gentiana lutea)*

Valerian root *(Valeriana officinalis)*
Vitamins
Minerals

Most of the above plants have a venerable history and, naturally
extravagant and poetic claims have been made:

> *   an essence of Balm, given in canary wine every morning will
>   renew youth, strengthen the brain, relieve languishing
>   nature and prevent baldness.

(from *The London Dispensary*, 1696)

Very little scientific work has been carried out on any of these
plants, so that their effect cannot be confirmed or denied in
this manner. It is as unlikely that they are useless as it is that
they will achieve some of the more spectacular results claimed.

Do Mild Remedies Work?

One might reasonably ask how these mild drugs of Chinese
therapeutics or of Western herbal medicine, are capable of
achieving anything at all. When many people realize that
medicinal plants such as ginger, cinammon, sage, lemon or
fennel are used as flavourings and spices, they cannot any
more regard them as medicinal. Even ginseng was used as a
condiment by the Chinese Emperors who would grate it onto
their breakfast like we might add wheat-germ to porridge, and
today the Koreans put ginseng into sweets, soup, flavourings,
chewing gum and bath essences, further devaluing it as a
therapy in the eyes of Westerners. This distrust of mild
medicaments is the basis for the distrust of practical herbal
medicine not of the value of medicinal plants as a whole, for it
is well known that many of our strong modern medicines are
derived from plants, such as digitalis from the foxglove.

As recently as last century, the botanicals were the only kind
of drugs, and were used both curatively and preventively.
Herbal preparations were often a matter of life and death,
particularly in disease prevention. The distrust of herbal
medicines has been gathering ground since the beginning of
the century. From that time onwards there has been a steady
decline in the reputation of herbals, in concert with the
glamour of the synthetic medicines, which are capable of
apparently instant cures of particular diseases such as

pneumonia, venereal diseases and so on. A glance at the annual series of National Pharmacopoiea shows that every year more and more herbals were dropped in favour of synthetic medicines, the replacement being more drastic in those countries actively researching and synthesizing new drugs. The herbals were dropped invariably without any evidence that they were useless. Today's attitude to mild herbs, 'old-wives' tales', is a result of the rise of a therapeutic system and a professional class who operate it, that promises instant cures. The herbs themselves have not changed. There are several reasons why mild herbs may be more effective than is commonly thought.

1. They are used in larger doses when necessary, certainly more than simply to impart flavour.
2. They are used under conditions which makes the body more sensitive to them. For example in the absence of stimulating drinks such as tea or coffee, tranquilizing herbs such as hops or passion flower are readily noticeable. Ginseng is more effective against a background of a light diet, sage will be more potent in drying up mucous in the absence of milk products in the diet. All herbs will be more effective in the absence of strong allopathic drugs in the body.
3. Herbs are taken consistently over a long period. This may mean simply a 2-week course. But it may also mean a lifetime during which herbs are consumed regularly.
4. They are often taken in cocktails or combinations in which various medicines affect and augment each other.
5. Timing is often important. With experience it is possible to determine the time of day, the season, or the stage of a disease, when herbs will be maximally effective.

5
GINSENG

As the Chinese have always claimed, ginseng could be a model remedy for the aged. Our non-mythical reading of traditional statements on ginseng makes it highly interesting and none the less mysterious. It may have restorative and protective abilities, but can this be proved scientifically? Does it relate to other known drugs or is it a radical departure from all our previous concepts of what drugs are like?

Traditional sources tell us more about ginseng that may help to fathom it. Firstly, that ginseng should not have any effect on a person already in perfect physiological harmony and health; its action is to return things to normal. Secondly, that it is particularly useful to those whose states of health are out of balance, especially in the direction of coolness, under-use, sluggishness and a build-up of toxins. Anaemic, convalescent, chronically ill, neurasthenic and exhausted people fall into this category, and of course the aged.

The long-term effects of ginseng use are extremely difficult to test using scientific methods. The latter have been developed during this century to test the curative effects of drugs on pronounced disease symptoms. There is little experience in the testing of tonic restorative or prophylactic (disease resisting) preparations, for they do not show any clear symptoms which might be corrected. How do you objectively ascertain if a person feels better? Or whether he is less likely to catch diseases? How do you study his future lifespan? It is even more difficult to ascertain the vitality of a mouse than a man, and although one can measure the lifespan and general health of mice it is tedious to do so. These problems mean that although some two thousand scientific papers have been published on ginseng, the experiments are often rather artificial, and limited in scope.

The first question is whether ginseng can be demonstrated to work at all, or whether it is a case of the well-known placebo effect, whereby an inert pill, given with words of encouragement can cause a significant improvement in health for purely psychological reasons. Of course, if this is a placebo effect, it means that four hundred million Chinese and countless Asians are all suffering from the giant illusion that ginseng is a medicine.

There have been occasional attempts to bring the 'wonder-root' into the laboratory ever since the beginning of the century. These resulted in a vague smattering of research results indicating that ginseng could adjust sugar metabolism and increase sexual activity and wakefulness in animals. In 1948 Professor Brekhman of the Far Eastern science centre of the USSR Academy of Sciences in Vladivostok started some experiments with ginseng. There was a range of plants with so-called tonic effects which Brekhman found in use in neighbouring China and Vietnam. He was fascinated by the possibilities of completely new kinds of medicinal properties in these plants and ginseng was the first to be put through its paces. Brekhman decided that it would be too difficult to test the general claims relating to health and vitality which the Chinese made for ginseng. Instead he reasoned that remedies that increased vitality ought to stave off exhaustion.

The first test was to give ginseng to 50 Soviet soldiers on a 3 km. race. Another 50 were given a similar tasting placebo, and neither knew who had the actual ginseng. The soldiers who had unknowingly taken the ginseng came in on average 53 seconds before the others. This was an extremely encouraging result. It was later successfully repeated with related plants, in particular *Aralia manshurica* and *Eleutherococcus senticosus*. Other scientists have repeated the study using pantocrine (deer horn extract) and found an average of 44 second improvement in times after a single dose, and a steady increase in performance as a result of long term administration. The experiments have been successfully repeated using an improved method of measuring physical stamina, a special kind of stationary bicycle.

This was not only the case with physical stamina. The Russians pioneered the use of text correction tests, proof reading tests, problem solving and morse code transmission by both professional and naive volunteers as a measure of mental energy, psychophysical coordination and efficiency. In the case of ginseng these tests have always given strongly positive results. For example, in the telegraphy tests the trained operators had to transmit two long hard texts. Those given the inert placebo made 28 per cent mistakes more in the second transmission while those given ginseng made 10 per cent *less* mistakes. Similar results have been obtained with other plants and with deer horn extracts. It is not only in the Soviet Union that these studies have been carried out. In an American study at the University of Minnesota, students did better in mock exams when they were given ginseng compared to placebo, although in this case the researcher did not notice much effect with *eleutherococcus*. At the Maudsley hospital in London we gave ginseng or identical placebo to nurses who were undergoing the strenuous and stressful change from daytime to night time work. We found that their performance in physical and psychological tests, their general level of mood, competence, energy, bodily symptoms, sleep time, and certain biochemical quantities were all reduced as a result of night work. Small doses of ginseng restored many of these aspects, particularly mood and competence scores. These experiments tell us that ginseng can improve arousal and human performance in conditions of exhaustion, and other related remedies can do likewise although they may be somewhat weaker.

Professor Brekhman summarizes his findings in this way:

> After a series of experiments on men it was established that daily doses of ginseng preparations during 15-45 days increase physical endurance and mental capacity for work. The increase was noted not only during the treatment itself, but also for a period of time (a month to a month and a half) after the treatment had been over. The increase in work capacity was attended by a number of favourable somatic effects and a general improvement of health and spirits (appetite, sleep, absence of moodiness, etc.)

These kinds of studies are much easier to do with mice. Mice also make such experiments more convincing, for it cannot be said that they have heard that ginseng is a panacea! A typical stamina test used to test stimulants and even anti-depressants, measures how long mice can swim in water, or climb a continuously moving rope, until complete exhaustion. Professor Brekhman found that in repeated trials his mice swam up to twice as long when they were given ginseng. In long term experiments, in which the mice were given ginseng and were made to swim regularly for thirty days, it was found that, as traditional Chinese sources have claimed, the effect of the ginseng built up over a period. At the end of the time the mice given ginseng swam for 96-117 minutes in comparison to 47-61 minutes for the others. Similar trials in London were successful using doses equivalent in mice terms to no more than those a man would take.

The existence of a simple test for ginseng has been of paramount importance, for it has enabled research workers to chemically analyse the ginseng root and test each component that they found. In this manner they have found that there are several anti-fatigue substances in the root. They are called ginsenosides in Japan and belong to a chemical group called *terpenoidal glycosides*. Their chemical nature is somewhat similar to steroids, which is an interesting discovery, for the steroids function as chemical messengers within our bodies. They are not all of equivalent strength. Other components have been isolated from the other Araliacea plants including *eleutherococcus* and they also perform in the laboratory in a similar manner to the whole plant. This is taken to mean that these components are the main, although not the only active compounds in the plants. When all the pharmacologically effective compounds of the various tonic Chinese plants are compared, one thing stands out: all of them, including the ginsenosides, are chemically related. They comprise a large group of similar substances which have never before been suspected of having interesting medicinal properties.

Homing In On Harmony

The discovery that the effects of ginseng can be objectively and repeatedly demonstrated in the laboratory opened the way for intensive explorations around the world which took off in a number of different directions. These are all described much more fully in *The Tao of Medicine*.

Investigation of the anti-fatigue properties are continuing mostly in Russia, but also in Japan and the University of California. These studies are going deeper into the way the muscles, the manufacturing and energy gathering processes, become more efficient during extended physical activity, when ginseng, *eleutherococcus* or their components are consumed. Several Soviet books and multitudes of papers have been published on these biochemical effects.

Another line of investigation has been to test animals for their ability to solve problems, learn, respond to cues, run around, sleep, and so on. The results, especially from scientists at Japanese Universities, indicate that small doses of ginseng help mice to learn and respond more readily. Indeed their performance in mazes was found to be better than when the mice had been given other classical stimulants such as amphetamine.

Now many drugs can increase learning ability and even stamina, such as caffeine or benzedrine. Ginseng is unrelated to these other drugs which are more toxic and act on the brain only. The difference is basically that ginseng type remedies restore energy while the stimulants squander it. As Brekhman puts it:

> Although ginseng is a powerful stimulant, it does not cause insomnia (if taken in therapeutic doses); its effects last longer, it does not, as does amphetamine, cause an initial decrease in work ability, and does not make one emotionally over-excited, as one so obviously gets with amphetamine. The stimulating effect of ginseng is especially noticeable during night watches, for example, in cases of extreme tiredness.

In the Soviet Union ginseng and *eleutherococcus* are used extensively in athletics, including at the recent Olympic games. This was under instructions from the sports authorities. The Russians find that their athletes have increased stamina and they adapt more easily during training.

All these studies tell us that ginseng makes more of an impact on exhausted and stressed animals or people than during their normal activity. We found this too at Chelsea College, University of London. Mice which had been given ginseng for a long time employed more exaggerated fear and avoidance motions when they were challenged, but when they were left alone did not alter their behaviour. Ginseng has a greater effect against a background of stress, and although the arousal effects of ginseng were recognized in traditional Chinese use, they were regarded merely as a spin-off of ginseng's restorative action.

Professor Brekhman explored this restorative activity more carefully by testing the survival of animals in the laboratory to a wide variety of stresses: chemicals such as drugs, poisons, alcohol or barbiturates; viruses, bacteria and the malaria parasite; diseases; or extremes of pressure and of temperature. In all cases they found a much greater chance of survival when ginseng or *eleutherococcus* were given to the animals.

Radiation was another stress used. The Russians found that double the number of animals could survive radiation if they were given ginseng first. We have confirmed in experiments at a Nuclear Research Centre, that ginseng can protect cells against radiation, and the Japanese have repeated the Soviet studies using mice, with essentially the same result.

The Russians were so impressed by their discovery that they began to give *eleutherococcus* widely to patients in Soviet hospitals who were receiving radiation treatment for cancer. Apparently the patients do not suffer so many devastating side-effects of such treatment. Moreover, there seems to be less chance for the cancers to re-seed in their body because of their improved resistance.

The resistance of the body to stress, danger or damage is controlled partly by the hormones of the adrenal glands. Some of these hormones, the *glucocorticoids*, activate various protective systems of the body. They recruit energy supplies, increase arousal and alertness, increase heart function, encourage the liver to remove poisons and mobilize the body reserves in readiness for the struggle. The adrenal glands are obviously a place to look for ginseng's action on the body. Researchers all over the world have now established that animals who have been given ginseng or *eleutherococcus* have a greater adrenal capacity to respond to stress. The glands produce the hormone more efficiently. As Dr Kim and his collaborators at Seoul University were first to show, the glands switch on more powerfully in the face of stress, and switch off more rapidly when the stress is passed.

The adrenal glands are in turn controlled by glands in the brain, which mastermind the body's reactions to the outside world. Professor Hiai of Japan has demonstrated that within fifteen minutes of the injection of ginsenosides into animals, the master glands in the brain begin to produce more hormone instructions. At Chelsea College, Professor Ginsberg, Deepak Shori and I have found that the brain becomes more sensitive to hormones that are involved in stress, when ginseng is given.

The importance of these studies arises from the fact that these hormones regulate internal harmony within the body. When a disturbance is threatened they activate the reactions by which the threat can be dealt with, without disruption or damage to the vital centres floating in their optimal internal world. If ginseng acts by making these hormonal reactions more efficient it would explain how it aids in resisting stress.

It goes further than that. For vitality can be seen as the energy and facility with which the organism deals with its world. If this interaction is made easier and more efficient, the organism becomes more vital as well as more resistant. For example, say that the environment is one of protracted coolness. An inefficient response would imply wastage of energy in heating the body and a less than perfect final temperature. Alternatively, if the environment is one of persistant noise and disturbance, an inefficient response would be to continuously pour out more hormones than are necessary and squander precious resources in a continual over-reaction. This state as we have seen, destroys health.

It seems as if ginseng and to some extent *eleutherococcus* are aiding the body in its fight to maintain a stable and harmonious internal state. That is why in an earlier publication I have termed these Chinese plants 'harmonizers', which is perhaps an improvement on the misleading term 'tonics'. The various properties which the ancient Chinese noticed, and which are also visible in the laboratory, such as increased alertness, stamina, adaptability, removal of poisons, improvement in the metabolic sources of energy, and so on, can all be understood as a result of actions on the control mechanisms of the body.

It is quite likely that many traditional plants which are

useful in health maintenance and vitality work in this kind of subtle fashion. For example, both liquorice and sarsaparilla, *Brahmi* and the chinese sage plant, have been shown in the laboratory to adjust hormones within the body. Even acupuncture has been demonstrated to produce alterations in the production of key regulatory hormones from the glands in the brain.

Just as a skilled mechanic will tune and service a car, adjusting parts which deviate and threaten a breakdown, so these adjustive medicines are employed in Chinese medicine to 'tune' the various body systems. The goal is harmony, and the means will differ according to the state of each individual. Different remedies suit each individual at that particular moment, in that particular environment. And just as a particular adjustment, say to the carburettor, will have differing effects depending on the state of all the other systems – the timing, the fuel grade, the valves, the spark plugs, etc. – so each remedy, ginseng included, will have differing effects on different people depending on their state of health at the time. This is why people have such a variety of reactions to the consumption of ginseng from an ecstatic burst of new life, to no effect at all, or even in rare cases to some unwanted side-effect. This may seem mysterious hocus-pocus to those well entrenched within the view of scientific medicine, in which each drug achieves a repeatable effect against each set of symptoms. However, in traditional medicine this variability is both expected and respected. For the traditional approach is state-specific. It deals with the whole individual who is seen as an animate slice of constantly adapting and interacting energy. Perhaps the reader can now understand why these adjustive remedies are regarded with such devotion by those who know how to employ them.

Ginseng, Poisons and Toxins

The accumulation of drugs, toxins or pollutants taken in from the world around each of us, is a serious constraint on health and longevity. Old people suffer especially from persistent toxins. In China, ginseng is specifically given to assuage side-effects of toxic and powerful drugs. One might suppose that ginseng could aid in removal of poisons since this is one of the functions controlled by the stress reaction mechanisms. Professor D. R. Hahn of the College of Pharmacy, Chung-Ang University, reports that ginseng helped the liver of mice to overcome damage by toxins such as *carbon tetrachloride* and *thioacetamide*. In another study, low doses of ginseng glycosides were given to experimental animals and then aspirin-type drugs injected. By measuring the quantities of these drugs in the blood at various times after administration, Professor Hahn and his colleagues found that the speed at which the drugs were removed was somewhat increased. In a parallel series of tests the rate of removal of alcohol from the blood was increased by about a third in animals given white ginseng and up to a half in animals given red root.

The Russians have found that *eleutherococcus* reduces both inebriation and the hangover. They market an eleutherococcus-vodka, which, they claim, is a healthier way to get drunk!

Sexual Function

Ginseng has a reputation as an aphrodisiac, mostly because of reports from the court of the Chinese Emperors in which it was used for that purpose. However, I believe that to claim that ginseng has specific aphrodisiac properties is a complete misreading of traditional usage. Ginseng is taken as a restorative. An important function which, in many people, is in need of restoration, is sexual capacity. Therefore in China, ginseng was taken in the hope of restoring sexual function by increasing general vitality. But to suggest that it is an aphrodisiac is as erroneous as to suggest that coffee is an examination-passing drug because people taking examinations drink lots of coffee. The day has not yet arrived when a safe long-term aphrodisiac is available, particularly as in most cases the problem is above the collar, not below the belt!

Nevertheless, there are studies showing that ginseng may have effects on the sexual glands, presumably as part of its overall effect on the hormones of the body. For example, one study reported that ginseng hastened the development of the prostate glands in young animals. In the Soviet Union *eleutherococcus* has been shown to improve the egg laying capacity of hens, and the fertility of various farm animals. While in Korea too, ginseng was shown to have significantly

increased the laying capacity of Hamphorn hens. The effect
was noticeable after several days of continuous administration
of small amounts. In another report ginseng appeared to
slightly reverse some of the changes produced by castration
to the tissues of the adult male laboratory rodent, and
Japanese scientists have reported an increase in sperm production in infertile men.

It is inconceivable that ginseng can turn the clock back and
restore full potency to older people who have lost sexual
capacity. On the other hand, there are enthusiastic claims by
the elderly men in China who are convinced that ginseng
allows them to father children in old age. As in so many cases,
the truth must lie somewhere in between the claims of the
healed and the scepticism of the experts.

Chinese Herbs, the Circulation and the Metabolism

In recent years Chinese doctors have dug up many herbal
preparations from the old Pharmacopaeia and tested them in
the modern city hospitals. Considerable success has been
reported in the use of such herbs in the treatment of heart
disease, an item of information which has not been lost to the
scientists of the National Institute of Health in America. For
example, one such plant is known as 'mao-tung-ching' (Ilex
pubescens), which belongs to the same genus as the holly. It has
been found to lower blood-pressure in patients with cardiovascular problems by dilating certain critical blood-vessels.
Ginseng has also been used in Chinese hospitals for the
treatment of heart conditions. A recent hospital trial of
ginseng compared it to Western medicines for the treatment of
low blood-pressure subsequent to heart attack. Ginseng
seemed to be able to stabilize the blood-pressure for a longer
period than the Western medicines.

Ginseng is widely used as a cardiac tonic in China. It is
valuable in cases of shock or after a heart-attack when the
blood-pressure has fallen, and the patient is in danger of heart
failure. Ginseng is given in mixtures where it usually adds an
energizing, balancing component to other more curative
remedies.

Ginseng might help in reducing blood-pressure, but its
effect is secondary and mild. In other words, its main use

would be to strengthen the body, and make it more efficient while other means were used to attack the blood-pressure problem directly. A German team of doctors reported that when they gave patients long term ginseng treatment, those with a systolic pressure above 140 showed an average drop measuring 23 millimetres. An elaborate study on the effect of ginseng on the circulation was published in 1964 from the Department of Pharmacology, University of Tenessee. Ginseng extract given to dogs produced an immediate drop in blood-pressure followed by a longer and milder increase, after which blood-pressure returned to normal.

In the USSR *eleutherococcus* is a regular component of treatment for high blood-pressure. It also tends to be widely distributed to workers in industrial environments as a preventative measure, to pre-empt stress induced increases in blood-pressure and cardiovascular deterioration. In the huge study at the Volga car works Dr Galanova found a reduced incidence of high blood-pressure compared to other workers in similar situations.

To summarize, ginseng and to a lesser extent *eleutherococcus,* can help the body to adjust abnormal blood-pressure. Ginseng raises low blood-pressure fairly rapidly and specifically. Its ability to reduce high blood-pressure is slow and limited and appears to be a secondary result of more general effects on the body.

The level of cholesterol in the blood is related to the production of hardening of the arteries. The amount of cholesterol is both the result of dietary factors and of stress-induced changes in body metabolism. Dr Hahn and other Korean scientists have shown that ginseng does reduce the amount of cholesterol in the blood of animals, and tends to convert it to fats which are stored, or to other components which are used up. The effect of ginseng in this regard is mild, and no result is noticed unless ginseng is given over a period of time. It is not too surprising that ginseng acts in this way since the processing of cholesterol, like blood-pressure, is stress-related.

In one study, for example, *ginseng saponin* was administered to animals for eight weeks during which time the cholesterol content of the blood decreased from 128.3 to 99.5 mg, while the cholesterol in the liver went down from 10.8 to 7.4 mg.

There was an adjustment in other fats. Trials of ginseng compared to other therapies were carried out on patients entering a Bahamas clinic. The doctor reported a drop in the cholesterol content in blood samples taken from patients on the ginseng therapy. However, in these cases it is rather difficult to distinguish the effect of ginseng from that of other factors in the environment of the patients, since all the patients received many treatments simultaneously.

Diabetes and its advance guard – high blood sugar, is also a disease of ageing, although it can sometimes occur in younger people. The amount of sugar in the blood, as with cholesterol, is the result of diet, exercise, arousal and other factors, regulated by several hormones. Ginseng has a reputation of normalizing or regulating blood sugar levels, presumably also through a hormonal mechanism. In a series of experiments reported in Russian, Chinese and Korean literature, ginseng has been shown to lower blood sugar levels, particularly when abnormally high. It cannot replace insulin in the management of diabetes, nor can it cure diabetes. When diabetes has occurred, most of the damage has been done and is not reversible. However, ginseng can assist in depressing blood sugar levels, as stated in one Chinese report, 'to produce a subsidiary effect in the treatment of the diabetic state'. Thus ginseng when intended for normalizing blood sugar, blood-pressure or blood cholesterol can be used in two ways. Either prophylactically, i.e. to prevent the onset of such diseases by regular but intermittent use, or to assist in the treatment of the diseases once they have occurred, in combination with curative medication, and appropriate dietary regimes.

Ginseng and the Elderly

Old people take ginseng seriously. One elderly, lady wrote to me that,

> I felt I must write and tell you of the wonderful effect the ginseng tablets have had on me. I have just passed my eightieth birthday and it is many, many years since I have felt so full of vitality and fitness as I have in the last few weeks. . . Usually I am sceptical of taking tablets recommended by other people because of unknown side-effects but there seemed no possible risk of this. I have been simply amazed at the improvement, not only in my physical

condition but also in the effect it has had on my mental alertness. Even the youngest members of my family have been convinced of its efficacy.

Our theoretical discussions in this chapter and our analysis of the traditional usage of ginseng would lead us to expect this kind of reaction from older people who start a course of ginseng. This is, after all, what a true restorative should do. But can we prove it? The problems involved in testing non-curative remedies in old people are immense. Nevertheless, a start has been made.

Most such studies have been carried out in European clinics or old age homes in which the patients or inmates were given a mixture of therapies which included ginseng. It is naturally difficult and sometimes impossible to separate the effects of ginseng from that of other treatments. For example, Dr Luth reported in *Ars Medici,* 1965, that he gave his geriatric debilitated patients a standard mixture containing, ginseng, vitamins and *dimethylaminoethyl.* At the end of one month he reported considerable improvement particularly in fatigu-ability, depression, and insomnia. He states that the preparation is 'suitable for counteracting the general falling-off in physical and mental abilities that is the first symptom of old age'. He later expanded his first sketchy analysis in a more extended test using, in addition to the previous mixture, a preparation containing all the constituents apart from ginseng. Neither the doctor nor the patients knew which preparation contained ginseng. It appeared that those patients taking the preparation containing ginseng showed improvements in mood, activity, interest and ability to sleep. Those taking the preparation without ginseng showed some improvement but not as much as the first group.

This early trial was limited because few patients were involved, and the analysis of health was highly subjective. A later study, carried out by Viennese doctors, attempted to provide a more authoritative review. Ninety-five patients in an old peoples' home took part, half receiving ginseng and half a placebo. The doctors noted improvements in the ginseng group in the quality and texture of the skin, as well as in blood flow in the small blood-vessels on the surface of the body. There was no change in breathing capacity, nor in the quality of the blood, but interesting results were obtained in blood-pressure measurements. Those with high blood-pressure showed a reduction of about 10 per cent, while the few patients with lower blood-pressure showed a rise of about 15 per cent. Appetite increased and 65 per cent of the patients gained weight while four overweight patients lost weight. 40 per cent of those patients suffering from insomnia were able to sleep better during the therapy. About the same number showed other improvements in nervous function such as co-ordination, steadiness, memory, and sense of balance. Mood changes were pronounced: 'Fifty-eight of the patients showed an enhancement of mood so marked as to be almost euphoric', write the authors, Drs Stengel and Listabarth. They found that the majority of patients showed increased initiative, increased desire to do things, increased pleasure from work, greater strength and stamina. There were improvements in the social environment and atmosphere, with two-thirds of the patients showing a better relationship with the staff of the home. As for tiredness, the doctors report that:

> it goes without saying that tiredness or exhaustion was one of our patients' main symptoms (83 cases out of 95). The psychological equivalent, manifesting itself as lack of desire to work, lack of participation, feeling of incapacity and of inability to concentrate, was included in these complaints. Sixty-nine patients, or 83 per cent showed clear improvements in both these syndromes, which can be considered an excellent result.

The course lasted for three months. The increases in activity and appetite could be seen after two to three weeks, and the other changes appeared thereafter. After the course the condition of a third of the patients deteriorated gradually to the old level and they began a new course. On the other hand, a quarter of the patients showed improvements which lasted for six months after cessation of the treatments. When the course of treatment was repeated the improvements apparently returned more quickly and lasted longer. The authors conclude that the preparation might be used as a 'prophylactic measure against disorders peculiar to old age'. A similar report by Dr Augusto Gianoli, Geriatric Consultant of the Tiefenan University Clinic in Bern, Switzerland, records that he has given this geriatric cocktail to more than six thousand patients for over ten years, with observation periods of between 6 months and 10 years. Again the author confirms the favourable effect of the preparation upon the health of his patients.

It must also be mentioned that there is at least one similar study which has been unable to obtain any conclusive information on whether or not the ginseng mixture is effective for older people.

These studies are only suggestive in relation to the effectiveness of ginseng since it is used in combination with vitamins and other components, some of which are known to affect the nervous system. There are, alas, hardly any trials with older people which test the effect of ginseng by itself. However, one such trial has been carried out in Italy and it distinguishes itself from all the others in the level of competence, fairness and accuracy with which it is carried out. This is a study at the Neuropsychiatric Hospital of the Province of Pavia. The authors gave three groups of patients different treatments. One received a standard preparation which is used to lower blood-pressure *(hydergine* – see below), together with the full ginseng, vitamin and DMAE mixture. Another received *hydergine* plus the mixture but without ginseng, and the third group, *hydergine* alone. In this way the authors hoped to be able to distinguish the effects of ginseng from those of the other components. The patients were examined, and given the various medicines for thirty days, at the end of which their health was examined again.

They found that the blood-pressure of the patients was similarly reduced in all three groups, and they found some relief of headache, insomnia, dizziness and speech problems. In this case too, there was no difference between the groups. This shows that neither ginseng nor the vitamin-DMAE complex has any advantages over *hydergine* in the control of blood-pressure, and the other functions. But distinct improvements were noticed in the control of the nerves and muscles in the body, measured by gait, mobility, tremble, weakness and ability to act independently. Here the mixture containing ginseng was about twice as effective as the other treatments.

Therapy was also successful in the psychological field. The elderly patients were initially severely handicapped by depression, loss of initiative, inability to act independently, poor memory and inability to concentrate. All the treatments produced major improvements, particularly the ginseng mixture. The authors stated that ginseng has an important part to play in the treatment of the decline in mental abilities during ageing, especially when combined with vitamins. Ginseng does not appear to have much effect on blood-pressure, or at least if it does, it is not more than that of *hydergine*, a special drug for reducing blood-pressure.

Perhaps the most careful and extensive study carried out so far has been performed by Dr U.J. Schmidt, head of the Gerontological Society of the DDR; 540 elderly patients were given ginseng extract, ginseng extract plus vitamins, or placebos. A massive test-battery of measurements was made. This included a minutely detailed medical, biochemical, neurological, psychiatric and psychological investigation. The researchers found that almost all of the subjective measurements of mood, drive, concentration and so on improved with the ginseng preparations as opposed to placebos. There was a significant drop in systolic blood-pressure (25 mm) in those whose blood-pressure was high, a drop in cholesterol levels, improved liver function and an especially noticeable improvement in the psychological tests measuring brain function, coordination, memory and ability to solve problems. The full results of this study are still awaited.

Ginseng and Lifespan

The claim that ginseng prolongs life is hard to test in man because the study would take so long that those carrying out the experiment would also be old at the end of it. Yet it is obvious that one can test whether or not ginseng can lengthen the lifespan of animals. It is only necessary to feed it to animals and measure how long they live. The first study to bring the longevity myths into the bright light of the laboratory in this way was carried out by the scientists of the Far East Scientific Centre. They gave ginseng to rats continuously after their mid-age, and recorded their subsequent lifespan. They found that ginseng was able to increase the average lifespan of their rats by 10 per cent. *Eleutherococcus* did somewhat better.

But nothing is so simple. The study did not use enough animals to produce reliable results and insufficient measurements were taken. More recently, I started a study of this type at Chelsea College, University of London, together with members of the Department of Human Biology. We used 270 mice, of which some were given ginseng continuously from birth, some from maturity and the rest were not given any treatment at all. The mice were carefully tended throughout their life and allowed to die naturally of old age. We used an amount of ginseng which would correspond to a normal human dose, and this was given in extract form and dissolved in their drinking water. We found that the mice in all three groups were healthy and active, and they weighed more or less the same. Ginseng did not, as far as we could judge, cause any harmful effects even when given from birth to death.

When all the lifespans of all the mice were measured it soon became clear that all the groups lived for roughly the same time, although there were certain minor differences. The average lifespan of female mice which had been given ginseng from birth was 90 weeks compared to 82 weeks for those mice which had not been given anything. The maximum lifespan of the female mice in the ginseng group was also slightly greater. However, these differences could possibly have happened by chance. The only point we felt confident about was that after ginseng had been given there was a period of several months when fewer mice than expected were dying. Clearly ginseng does not dramatically affect the lifespan of mice under these conditions. That is not to say that giving ginseng in a different way or in a different dose may not have had a greater effect. However, it does confirm our view that the common cultivated ginseng by itself, is not the life prolonging elixir that the folk tales suggest.

Scientific research with older people has confirmed that ginseng can produce increased vitality during ageing. Energy is the key to a healthy old age. It brings with it benefits for the psyche such as confidence, morale, contentment and involvement. These in turn save the body because of a reduction in stress and tension, greater resistance and increased exercise. Extra years might follow, particularly if health was developed through an appropriate life style. But it would be a gain in lifespan that would not necessarily reveal itself in these kinds of experiments.

The traditional experience that ginseng 'harmonises energies... removes toxic substances... strengthens the soul...

and invigorates the body' have now been supported by scientific research. Other claims, such as 'repairing the yang' cannot yet be approached, given the language and methodology of science. However, there is proof enough that ginseng and its close relatives are of special relevance to the aged. Old people tend to be more vulnerable, suffer from stress- related conditions, are colder, more easily tired, more sluggish in metabolism and the removal of toxins. These are the very states which are aided by ginseng.

Taking Ginseng

For those who want to try ginseng the following guidelines can be drawn up. These are based on a synthesis of the advice of traditional sources in countries with a history of ginseng use. They apply to the conditions likely to be met in the West. However, everyone responds somewhat differently, so that no rigid recommendations can be made.

1. Quality.
Panax ginseng: First quality are large red roots from Korea or China. The best are six years old, and they decline in quality and price in proportion to size and age. Second quality are large white roots from Korea or China. These too decline in quality according to size and age. Third quality and a poor third at that, are red roots grown in Japan and boxed in a somewhat similar manner to top quality Korean red roots to confuse the customer. They do not, however have the Korean 'Office of Monopoly' seal on them.
The whole roots are always best, followed by pieces of root, followed by extracts. Ginseng powder or tablets are next in quality because they are often bulked out at source with inert material. The lowest grade are the instant ginseng teas, which contain hardly any active constituents.

Panax quinquefolium: The American ginseng can sometimes be obtained wild, in which case it probably equals *Panax ginseng* in effectiveness. However, most American ginseng is cultivated and it is less effective than *Panax ginseng* from Asia. Again, the oldest and largest roots are always the best.

Eleutherococcus senticosus: (Siberian ginseng) is best bought as original extract from the USSR which is guaranteed pure.

Failing that, one can find tablets from reputable firms. Avoid it if it has *Acanthopanax sessiliflorum* on the packet.

2. Dosage

The dosage is not fixed, but dependent on a person's needs, state of health, constitution, age, diet and also on the type of root. The dosages given below are for average white whole cultivated roots. A dose of 1-2 g per day would be an average long term restorative dose for adults. The dose can be increased during convalescence, or during the treatment of the various conditions for which ginseng is useful. The Koreans recommend about 4 g per day in such cases. For short-term intermittent use, for example when particularly tired or stressed, the dose can also be increased. Older people can also take more if they feel it helps. Less ginseng need be taken by particularly sensitive people or those on various controlled diets, in particular vegetarians. For extracts or teas, dosage instructions cannot be given here since the amount of ginseng varies in different preparations. The product literature should be referred to in these cases.

3. Period

To make the most of ginseng it should be taken regularly over some time. An average period would be one month, although this often depends as much on an individuals' pocket as on anything else, and there are no hard and fast rules. For younger people it would be best to take such a course only once or twice a year, preferably in the autumn or winter. In China, the older people take it as often as possible, preferably continuously, and there is no reason why anyone above the age of menopause should not do likewise. Ginseng can also be taken intermittently when needed, either as a short-term tonic or to cope with unusual stresses or demanding situations, however this manner of usage of ginseng will not contribute to long-term health.

4. Conditions and Precautions

Women should, in general, *not take Panax ginseng*, but rather *Eleutherococcus sentocosus* (Siberian ginseng) unless they are above the age of menopause when they can take *Panax ginseng.* Anyone who gets a headache or feels over-excited when taking ginseng should reduce the dose or switch to *Eleutherococcus*. People with very high blood-pressure should not take *Panax ginseng* unless recommended by their practitioner. Younger people should avoid caffeinated drinks (tea or coffee) while taking ginseng, which would spoil the benefits and possibly lead to insomnia. It should not be taken by younger people in spring or summer. It should *not* be taken along with *Vitamin C* or any steroid treatment.

In order to extract the maximum benefit from a course of ginseng, it is advisable that the diet be limited. This means in particular that meats and heavy foods be avoided, and food consumption reduced. You might feel more energetic and lively during the course of ginseng, although not everyone does so. It would be a mistake to utilize this extra energy for the purpose of rushing about madly and becoming more stressed than normal. It stands to reason that if ginseng can assist in stress adaption, this advantage will be lost if it is merely used to pile on further stress. For long-term benefit, a course of ginseng must be accompanied by rest and a reduction in stressful situations. It must be approached with an attitude of taking a holiday. It would be useful to combine it with other exercises towards health. The Chinese also recommend celibacy during a serious ginseng course.

6
ALLOPATHIC ALTERNATIVES

Traditional remedies are usually mild, safe and effective. Yet there may be problems connected with their use. The most serious derives from the fact that they need be taken as part of a therapeutic milieu. But the competent, sensitive and individual advice which is required is to build a programme of health restoration around these remedies is not always available. The scarcity of expertize is due to the overwhelming dominance of our conventional medical system. A second problem is that there are inadequate supplies of traditional remedies, and sometimes they are of poor quality and high price. A third problem is that it is not always easy to go against the grain, especially for elderly people – to use 'folk' remedies despite the ridicule and incomprehension of friends, relatives or doctors.

What about modern drugs? We cannot assume that they are all just curative and damaging to long-term health. Nor can we assume that traditional and folk practitioners have a monopoly on longevity remedies. For these reasons it is important to search for synthetic or chemical drugs which might also be of relevance to us. Which substances might a doctor prescribe to the elderly?

Here, too, we are not concerned with curative drugs – remedies, however mild, which relate to specific conditions. There are harmless medicines within the allopathic sphere, such as laxatives, which may be of considerable help to some people via an action on some specific body system. However, since they are not directly related to ageing or the question of vitality and general health, they do not concern us here.

Remedies to Avoid

Before considering possible useful chemical remedies, let us consider certain drugs which are frequently given to older people and which cause a great deal of harm. These are drugs which might be given by doctors to older people who are tired, feeling the effects of their age, chronically depressed and resigned and full of vague and changing symptoms and discomforts. The doctor will not prescribe a curative drug, since there is no diagnosable specific disease entity. But he might prescribe certain other classes of drugs which are often unnecessary. These remedies may switch off the complaints, but they may also switch off health. They are given in place of personalized health restorative instruction which few doctors have the time or ability to provide.

One of the more serious drugs given to older people is cortisone. It is a complaint stopper in that it can reduce the overall level of symptoms, particularly when they include allergies, arthritis or skin problems. However, it only acts on the symptoms and the general feeling of well-being associated with cortisone is temporary. General resistance and vitality are reduced, the body's metabolism and water balance are unnecessarily altered. It makes health restoration more difficult.

Among the kaleidoscopic array of tablets and preparations found in the medicine cabinet of today's older person, the most common are the drugs which affect the nervous system. Many elderly people suffer from depression and insomnia, which may be a consequence of reduced physical activity, discomfort and lack of vitality, as well as psychological factors. Sleeping pills such as barbiturate derivatives are prescribed heavily in Western countries. Sleeping preparations all have prolonged effects which last over the night and well into the next day, causing tiredness, confusion or fogginess. Many experts feel that they are far too easily handed out by medical authorities when proper sleep might be obtained through a change in life-style, diet, or activity patterns. The easy availability of sleeping pills causes many to be desperately and needlessly reliant on them for a good night's sleep. The extensive use of sleeping pills will add to other factors in reducing vitality and should be avoided where reasonably possible.

The same applies to drugs acting against depression. There are, of course, cases of depression where urgent medication is necessary so that the individual can lead some sort of normal life. But these drugs are usually symptomatic, that is they may merely remove the feeling of depression, but the underlying causes will still exist. Most of the antidepressant drugs are taken by people with mild but continuous depression who would probably benefit from changing their habits, foods and pattern of living as much as from taking toxic antidepressant drugs. These drugs have generally more serious side-effects than sleeping pills, especially in older people. The commonest type, termed the tricyclic antidepressants, can also cause sedation and fogginess. They have the added problem of possible effects on the cardiovascular system, and they interact and alter the effects of other drugs. Other antidepressants, termed the MAO inhibitors, have the possibility of even worse side-effects. The problems of depression and insomnia are more easily assisted by changes in activity and life-style, than most of the other complaints from which older people suffer.

Tranquillizers are also frequently supplied to the elderly. They are specifically given for anxiety, hypochondria, stress diseases such as gastric ulcers, tension, agitation and distress. The most common tranquillizers are the *Valium* or *Librium* type. However, here again the drugs only affect the symptoms and the root causes are left untouched. Indeed, anxiety is sometimes caused by a continuous feeling of being one degree under. In this case it is obviously health and vitality which should be attended to, and with that improved, the anxiety may also be relieved. A treatment which simply suppresses the symptoms of worry is not treatment at all. Tranquillizers have side-effects which are subtle but are certainly very prolonged. They may make the search for positivity and vitality more difficult. Tonic remedies cannot replace such drugs, but when combined with healthy living could improve underlying physical and mental causes of the anxiety symptoms for which tranquillizers are intended.

Another very common group of drugs are those which reduce blood-pressure and strengthen the heart, and their frequency indicates the collossal scale of cardiovascular problems in industrial societies. Unfortunately, these drugs have profound side-effects. One report indicated that 60 per cent of men taking a typical preparation for reducing blood-pressure became impotent. These drugs frequently produce depression and in older people certain types may in the long run cause more heart problems. They can also interact with other types of drugs such as certain antidepressants. The picture is a sorry one, since by the time the blood-pressure is high enough to risk medication, most of the damage has been done.

Older people cannot neutralize and remove drugs as easily as the young. A younger person can flush toxic drugs out of his system, whereas in an older person they may persist and interact with one another. The older person is anyway more vulnerable to damage or upset, and will tend to slip into genuine disease states more easily than with the young. An Australian study reported that some 12 per cent of the old people in hospital are there as a result of the side-effects of drugs.

Bearing this in mind, let us now consider modern drugs and food supplements which could be useful in arriving at a healthy old age.

Vitamins and Minerals

Vitamins were discovered because certain foods could cure deficiency diseases. For example Vitamin C, ascorbic acid, was discovered because it was known that something in limes or lemons could prevent scurvy. Similarly with Vitamin D and rickets, iodine and goitre, iron and anaemia. Since the vitamins were discovered in this way, it was a logical step to define the amounts needed in the diet as that quantity which would prevent the deficiency diseases. In the case of Vitamin C this is 60 mg a day for a human. The deficiency disease system of calculating doses is characteristic of the methods of our disease oriented medical system. A health-oriented medical system would instead ask how much vitamin is needed to maintain your peak health. In the case of Vitamin C, the answer is some 10 to 100 times higher than the minimum scurvy preventing dose. Indeed the dose of vitamin C needed to keep monkeys healthy, based on their diet in the wild, recommended by the U.S. Committee on Animal Nutrition is some 60 times greater than the Recommended Daily Allowance for humans!

We require a large number of vitamins and minerals. Sufficient will usually be obtained by a varied and natural diet to avoid any signs of deficiency and provide a minimum basis for health. If processed, stored or refined foods are eaten then deficiencies are easily possible, either because the diet does not include them, or because such foods interfere with their absorption. For example a meat and white bread based diet will have insufficient vitamin E, some B vitamins, vitamin C, calcium and other minerals; eating white sugar can lead to a magnesium deficiency. Eating a natural and balanced diet is obviously the first requirement for health and provides the basis upon which to add special remedies related to ageing. Diet is discussed elsewhere in this book. Therefore we will only discuss here those vitamins and minerals which might need to be taken as supplements or remedies in relation to ageing, in addition to those received by an adequate diet.

The use of larger doses of certain vitamins is justified by the fact that some of them have protective roles in the body and it is possible to increase general health by their use. In addition, they can adjust metabolic processes in a favourable direction. For example, large doses of niacin, (vitamin B_3), can improve and stabilize the sugar metabolism of the body, restoring carbohydrate imbalances in alcoholics and people suffering from low blood sugar. Vitamins have an important role in preventing premature ageing and possibly in extending the lifespan.

Vitamin C

Vitamin C is one of the most important vitamins to take as a supplement. It has an important protective role in the body, and there is good evidence that increasing vitamin C dosage above that obtained from fruit and vegetables in the diet, can have a beneficial effect on general health. Vitamin C has been found to protect the body from infectious diseases, especially cold and 'flu, by bolstering natural defences. It aids in the healing of wounds, prevention of kidney and bladder-stones and possibly of diseases such as rheumatism, arthritis, cancer, circulatory diseases, hepatitis and others. It may also help in convalescence and recovery.

Vitamin C assists the body in detoxifying and removing poisons, especially some metals, and may thus be especially important in the polluted world in which we live. Similarly, it assists in maintaining the correct levels of cholesterol and in the removal of the breakdown products of fat metabolism. One of its functions in the body is to assist in the manufacture of certain hormones from the adrenal glands, hormones which have an important function in protecting the body from stress and damage. It is thus needed in extra amounts to overcome episodes of stress.

Vitamin C is one of the body's natural 'anti-oxidants'. That is, substances which assist in preventing the materials of the body from deteriorating in a manner similar to the browning of bruised fruit or the creation of rancidity in fats. This decomposition is chemical rather than bacterial and is brought about by oxygen in the air and by internal 'oxidative' chemical breakdown. Vitamin C acts like anti-oxidants which are added to foods to stop them spoiling. One of the current theories of the cause of the ageing process is that it is due to insidious and inexorable oxidation of essential biological polymers. The oxidation proceeds through the creation of 'wild' molecules called 'free radicals', which are powerful oxidizers. Free radicals have been shown to produce an oxidative destruction which increases with age. They affect collagen, one of the main structural proteins of the body, leading to toughening of the tissues, inflexibility of blood-vessels, wrinkling of skin and other ageing-type signs. Free radicals in the body are increased by radiation, pollutants, some heavy metals (e.g. lead), ozone, nitrites, and possibly even toxic residues resulting from exhaustion, stress or illness. This is one way in which these substances may accelerate ageing. Antioxidants and some free radical removing substances have been found to prolong the life of animals in the laboratory.

Vitamin C is an effective free-radical removing substance. It 'scavenges' the body for these agents and neutralizes them. At the same time it stops oxidative decay. Therefore, it may be quite important as an ageing-protective agent when taken regularly throughout the lifespan. This is particularly true when individuals are affected by poor diets, stress, toxins and pollution.

The dosage of vitamin C is in dispute. Some say 1 g a day, others up to 15 g. At the highest dosage, problems may occur. A safe average dosage might be 1 g a day plus whatever was consumed in food. The best way of taking it is probably in month long courses with breaks in between. The dosage can be temporarily increased in situations of risk, poisoning or stress.

Vitamin E

Vitamin E is another strong anti-oxidant and protective agent. It is a collection of oily compounds and is therefore particularly important in neutralizing the deterioration of body fats and oils. It is naturally present in unrefined vegetable oils, nuts and seeds and is sometimes taken in the form of wheat-germ oil.

Vitamin E assists in the synthesis of factors related to energy metabolism. It prevents the collection and deposition of cholesterol in the arteries. Vitamin E also protects hormones and certain vital substances from deterioration and adds to the anti-oxidant effects of other anti-oxidants such as Vitamin C. In fact vitamin C can restore vitamin E which has been chemically exhausted.

Soviet experiments have been carried out using large doses of vitamin E and vitamin A. Ageing people given this cocktail were reported to improve in strength, sleep quality, and the appearance of skin and hair. However, it is not clear whether the subjects were prematurely aged in the first place, a question which complicates rejuvenatory experiments. Studies with animals have failed to show substantial lifespan prolonging effects with vitamin C or vitamin E but moderate extensions have been recorded in mice and flies. However, it is not known if the animals were perfectly healthy and would anyway live out their maximum lifespan. We can conclude from this that like vitamin C, vitamin E has a protective role in preventing premature ageing, particularly that resulting from stress, poisons, pollution or chronic disease. These vitamins can evidently help to ensure a healthy old age although they are not elixirs of life.

Vitamin E supplemental dosage is also a matter of debate and advice should be obtained. For example, the more fat that is consumed, the more vitamin E should be taken. Doses of 200 International Units per day in total is regarded by some nutritionists as optimum. However, people with diabetes, high blood-pressure or other diseases should consult their practitioner about vitamin E dosage.

Other vitamins such as vitamin A, B, D vitamins, folic acid and choline, all have their role to play in maintaining health, although none are so relevant to a healthy old age as C and E. Of the large group of B vitamins, perhaps niacin (B_3) and pantothenic acid (B_5) are of most importance. Niacin has been found to reduce fatty deposits in skin and arteries and to counteract blood clotting, while B_5 is involved in the synthesis of various compounds needed for energy metabolism and brain function. B_5 has been reported to be one of the main components of royal jelly. Supplements of B_5 have increased the lifespan of laboratory animals on an otherwise adequate diet by 20 per cent.

Extra B vitamins can be recommended in periods of stress. However, it is difficult to recommend supplements of individual B vitamins and the other vitamins on a regular basis throughout the lifespan since this could lead to paranoid and excessive vitamin pill consumption without adequate justification. The sensible course would be to ensure more than adequate supplies of B and D vitamins through the consumption of yeast, wheat germ and other vitamin rich and natural foods, and reserve supplementation for times of stress. However, during old age itself reasonable supplementation with multivitamins can be unhesitatingly recommended.

Minerals

Minerals are just as important in their way as vitamins, however, they play a different part in body function. They are usually required as essential components of certain body tools called enzymes. A proper varied natural diet should provide a minimum of all the minerals necessary. However, there are one or two which might be considered for supplementation in relation to ageing.

Selenium is an essential mineral which is also involved in the antioxidative and detoxification processes of the body. It complements vitamin E by affecting its distribution in the body. Selenium varies in the diet, depending on its concentration in the particular geographical area upon which the food is grown or the livestock reared. There is some epidemiological evidence that high selenium intake is associated with lower incidence of certain cancers, particularly breast cancer, as well as heart diseases. Selenium is taken as a supplement by some longevity-minded Americans, usually at a dose of ¼ mg a day. The best way to take it is through brewer's yeast which has been grown in a selenium – containing broth.

Most of us eat too much salt. One of the key causes of heart problems is an excess of sodium, derived mostly from dietary salt (sodium chloride). There should be a balance of sodium and potassium in the body, and persistent dominance of sodium is a serious danger to health in the long term. Balance can be achieved by reducing salt in the diet, eating fruit and avoiding processed and refined foods.

Zinc is related to ageing. It is required for the synthesis and manipulation of vital informational molecules in the body, and in renewal of tissues. It may be involved in the prevention of age-related arthritic disease. More important, it can neutralize excess copper in our diet, by balancing the copper in the tissues. Zinc can also displace cadmium, an unwanted and toxic metal, from our tissues.

There is a good deal of evidence that copper can add to causative agents in hardening the arteries, in increasing the oxidative deterioration of fats and in hastening senility. Excess copper is quite common in our tap water.

Unwanted minerals, particularly lead, aluminium, copper, cadmium, mercury and bismuth are a bane of modern life. They are pervasive; present in tap water, air, dust and polluted foods and cooking utensils. There is evidence that they can hasten mental deterioration with age and shorten lifespan. Aluminium, for example, has been found in much higher levels in the brains of aged people with senile dementia than others of the same age. Even small amounts of lead and mercury produce confusion and mental deterioration. There are basically three ways of dealing with these metals:

1. To avoid consuming them as much as possible. For this purpose it is usually necessary to determine the quality of the local tap water and consider substitutes. Besides diet, it is wise to be aware of the problem of polluted air in inner city areas and near main roads. Do not use aluminium or pervious pans.
2. To use purification procedures. Vitamin C will assist in the removal of these minerals. Occasional fasting removes some accumulated toxins including metals.
3. To displace them from the body by including the correct minerals in sufficient quantities in the diet. Calcium displaces lead, zinc – copper, selenium – mercury.

Nucleic Acids and Cell Therapy

Nucleic acids are the inner sanctum of all living tissues, the constituents which transcribe, reproduce and direct all our living functions. They are long chains of molecules on which instructions are encoded like a computer tape containing morse code. Ever since nucleic acids were discovered, scientists have intuitively felt that here lies the key to ageing. It has been a favourite pastime of most ageing theorists to involve nucleic acids in concepts about the nature and origin of ageing. Indeed, perhaps the most important theory of the origin of ageing is that ageing occurs through the gradual and cyclic production of mistakes in the informational systems of the cell.

Experiments have been carried out in which nucleic acids were fed to animals to see if they lengthened life. Small but consistent increases in the lifespan have been obtained. However, the reason for this is uncertain as nucleic acids are dismembered by digestive processes and one cannot therefore pass any 'youthful' information into an organism in that way. Perhaps the provision of extra nucleic acid building blocks may add useful metabolic components, facilitating cell division, repair and so on. The consumption of food such as yeast, lentils, fish roe and small fish such as sardines, will add nucleic acids to the diet. This is the basis of 'Dr Frank's No-Ageing Diet' which recommends 2 g of dietary nucleic acid a day. This would seem on the high side (3 tablespoonsful of yeast would provide 1 g), and might even cause gout in sensitive individuals. The claims made by him and by the school are exaggerated. Consumption of some nucleic acid-rich foods can do no harm but their effects on ageing are unproven.

Several European doctors have taken a more logical step in giving their patients injections of nucleic acids. There is evidence that tissues and cells do take up entire nucleic acid molecules and incorporate source of their information. Nucleic acids are obtained from different organs of animals, plus some from yeast. It is hoped that the nucleic acid from each organ will rejuvenate the same organ in the person to whom it is given. Anecdotal and subjective reports from the doctors concerned speak of profound improvements in general health of prematurely aged individuals, and increases in memory and brain function in most patients. This treatment is expensive and restricted to some European doctors who are interested in rejuvenation.

A better known rejuvenatory procedure was developed by a Swiss surgeon, Paul Niehans, which he termed 'cell therapy'. The logic behind it is reasonable although there is considerable controversy over whether it actually works. In 1931 Niehans was called upon to attempt to save a woman whose parathyroid gland had been damaged. He was unable to save the gland surgically but instead hit on the last resort idea of injecting parathyroid cells obtained from an animal. The woman was cured and lived on into her nineties. He began to use this method as a substitute for organ transplantation in those people with damaged or deteriorated organs.

The aspect of this work that baffles and rebuffs the experts is that Niehans claims that the normal processes by which the body rejects 'foreign' materials does not reject these cells. This may be partly due to the use of cells derived from sheep foetuses. At the foetal stage cells do not have such characteristic signals by which the immunity of the person into whom they are injected can recognize their foreignness. Nevertheless, it is still a puzzle to experts, many of whom feel that the cells must be destroyed in some way, perhaps slowly, which would invalidate the procedure. However, for Niehans the lack of evidence of destruction of his cells opened the floodgates to the use of this procedure for all kinds of diseases and problems, as well as rejuvenation. For example, for heart diseases he would inject the cells of a young sheep's heart. For impotence he would inject the cells of the sexual glands, as well as the glands in the brain, which make hormonal triggers for sexual activity. For rejuvenatory purposes he would inject cells from several organs at different times, concentrating particularly on the organs manufacturing hormones.

Hormones are critically important in controlling the health and balance of the body. When hormones decline in accuracy, efficiency and responsiveness, the entire physiology of the body is thrown out of kilter. It is now fairly well established that the function of the hormone glands can pace the ageing process – early deterioration of the glands producing early ageing. This is especially true of the master glands, the hypothalamus and pituitary, which have a cascade of influences on other hormone glands and organs in the body.

While many people have suggested that consuming the hormone glands of younger animals might rejuvenate the glands of older people, of course this has never been possible. This is because the digestive process breaks down animal products to a soup of degraded molecules. It is also impossible to graft younger organs because of the problem of graft rejection. All this did not stop hormone glands being used in traditional medicine– the placenta, the testes and even semen were classical medicines in China. Some of the smaller hormones from these glands would pass through the gut, however rejuvenation was not actually expected from these traditional animal medicines.

We have already mentioned the futile maverick efforts of Brown-Sequar with his testicular injections. His disciple, Voronoff, made a fortune from the testicular grafting of monkey testicles on to those of the wealthy. The result was a great deal of suffering and poor health when the grafts failed to take. The descendant of all these efforts is the use of oestrogen and testosterone in modern medicine to cope with symptoms arising from hormonal and sexual decline. No-one can claim, however, that these externally administered hormones provide long term rejuvenation.

Niehans may have developed the best method for the incorporation of young hormones into the bodies of aged people. He may indeed be able to get round the graft rejection problem. Thousands upon thousands of people, including at least one recent Pope, have taken his injections in various European clinics. Injectable cells are now prepared in modern pharmaceutical laboratories. Yet it is highly unlikely that profound rejuvenatory results can be obtained in the case of normal healthy people. A temporary prolongation of certain functions may be possible, perhaps for longer than by injection of hormones by themselves, but not general rejuvenation. The main importance of Niehans' procedure may be to those who senescence is premature or who suffer from deterioration of sexual or other functions as a result of an early or precipitous decline in hormone production.

Novel Chemicals

The school of gerontologists who believe that our demise is largely due to run-away oxidation of our tissues have a handy solution: food preservatives. Such substances are added to foodstuffs to preserve them from oxidation while in storage. Preservatives such as BHT *(butylated hydroxytoluene), ascorbyl palmitate, ethoxyquine, sodium bisulphite* and a multitude of others are regarded by many as one of the main sources of contamination of our foods and a dangerous commercial practice. Yet several scientists believe that certain of these chemicals, in appropriate dosages are not only harmless, but also promote longevity!

The campaigners for these preservatives state that such substances have not been shown to produce any harmful effects in dosages much higher than their permitted maximum in foods. The lethal dose of BHT or BHA in humans is, of course, unknown. But from animal tests it would appear to be some 100-200,000 times the actual daily dose in the average American diet. BHT in quite high quantities, has been given to animals during their life. An extraordinary 50 per cent increase in lifespan has been reported. Denham Harman at the University of Nebraska compared the life extension of various anti-oxidants fed to normal mice. 8.7 per cent of the untreated mice lived to 20 months while 6.1 per cent of the mice fed BHT, 74.6 per cent of the mice fed *ethoxyquine,* and 13.2 per cent of the mice fed vitamin E lived to 20 months. Considerable increases in lifespan of mice fed *ethoxyquine* have also been found in experiments in the U.K. Added to this,

BHT has been found to greatly reduce the incidence of gastrointestinal cancers in strains of mice particularly vulnerable to such cancers.

These experiments have provided sufficient reason for some ardent American longevists to take up to 1 g of these food preservatives a day dissolved in oil. However, it would seem premature to take these chemicals before it is known if subtle long-term detrimental effects occur. While none has been found in animals on quite high doses, it does not mean that humans will be immune from side-effects. Indeed, there is no evidence that humans can actually increase their lifespan in this way and none is likely to be forthcoming in the near future. One of the main problems with extrapolating from mice studies to man is that mice are housed under artificial laboratory conditions and are genetically inbred. Their lifespans may be compromised in the first place, and then restored by additives such as BHT in the food. If that is the case the evidence supporting the use of these additives vanishes.

Amygdalin, also called vitamin B_{17} or laetrile is a notorious chemical related to cyanide, that has been claimed to both prevent and cure cancer. It is the brain child of a U.S. biochemist by the name of Krebs, who claims that it not only can cure cancer in some cases, but it can also prevent certain ageing diseases such as atherosclerosis and cirrhosis of the liver. It is present in small amounts in seeds, grains and legumes, and in much larger quantities in apricot kernels. A dose of about 20 kernels a day is recommended. The theory behind the use of amygdalin in both prevention and cure is that it is taken up by potential cancer cells which thereby destroy themselves. There is evidence both for and against amygdalin and it is the subject of furious controversy in America. The U.S. Food and Drug Administration has banned the sale of pure amygdalin. Perhaps the best support for it is based on traditional folk wisdom of the longevous people of the Hunza and generally in the Middle East, which regards apricot kernels as a preventive remedy.

We should mention certain sulphur-containing substances. They are also involved in protecting the body from oxidative processes, particularly the formation of crosslinks which harden and wrinkle structural proteins. One substance, called cysteamine is a classical radiation protecting material and has been found to radically restore the immune (disease prevention) system of older animals, in very reliable experiments performed at the U.S. National Institute of Health. Other sulphur containing materials are used to protect and restore wrinkled skin and capture and remove contaminating heavy metals, such as lead. Sulphur containing compounds such as cysteine and methionine are naturally occurring in our bodies, and join with other sulphur containing compounds in eggs and especially in garlic. Since some vegetable proteins, such as that of beans, are poor in sulphur-containing compounds, it would be advisable for vegetarians to eat plenty of garlic or an occasional free-range egg. Some people take supplements of cysteine, methionine or other sulphur compounds, especially if they are strict vegetarians.

The Procaine Panegyric?

When Sigmund Freud promoted the virtues of cocaine at the end of the last century he unwittingly prepared the way for the most famous of all ageing remedies. Freud and others first applauded the use of cocaine as a completely effective and yet reversible local anaesthetic. It was a revolutionary discovery. However, they soon reluctantly became aware that cocaine was addictive. A search for safe substitutes began and procaine was synthesized at the turn of the century. It could anaesthetize nerves in the areas where it was injected, yet within a few minutes the procaine was rendered inert by the tissues, and the nerves recovered their sensations. Procaine is not addictive and not toxic.

Soon after it was discovered, some observant European doctors noticed that arthritic patients derived considerable benefit from procaine injections. It became a classical antiarthritic until it was eclipsed by the discovery and manufacture of cortisone, the 'miracle drug'. During the Second World War, a Rumanian professor Parhon, and his assistant, Dr Ana Aslan, found that patients receiving procaine injections appeared to feel and look younger, they had a reduction in other symptoms such as those of circulatory deterioration, and some, apparently, enjoyed a return of their hair colour.

Ana Aslan opened a clinic in Rumania and she treated people for chronic degenerative diseases including atherosclerosis, nervous disorders, arthritis and asthma. However, her main claim was in respect of severe or premature ageing symptoms. She used as a primary treatment, frequent injections of a procaine preparation which contained added stabilizers, which she called *Gerovital*. She repeatedly stated that the treatment was long-term, and no changes could be expected in less than four months.

Patients flocked to her clinic. It attracted world-wide attention. Famous people, such as Charlie Chaplin, took cures there, and her patients developed a fanatical loyalty to her. Meanwhile, she campaigned ceaselessly for the rejuvenatory possibilities of procaine. Soon it became available to doctors in Europe as a preparation termed KH3 and began to be widely used, and at this point the medical world in western countries began to sit up and take notice.

The medical establishment was in general derisive and caustic. They were looking for cast iron evidence of anti-ageing effects. All Ana Aslan was able to provide was many anecdotal and subjective reports, and an almost obsessive and uncritical promotion of procaine, a stance that could hardly endear her to European researchers. An editorial appeared in the *British Medical Journal* of 1959 which voiced the prevalent view that procaine is certainly an excellent local anaesthetic, and it may be a reasonable anti-arthritic, and it could, conceivably, produce skin changes in some cases, but that there was absolutely no evidence, as far as they could ascertain, that procaine had anything to do with the symptoms of ageing or other diseases. Their view was bolstered by a series of clinical trials in the U.K., using demented, aged patients in institutions, who showed no effects from the procaine. Aslan herself refused to carry out clinical trials. She felt that clinical trials, which need comparative groups of people who do not receive the medication, were unethical.

Aslan declared that the previous trials used inadequate dosages for too short a time, with patients who were far too senile to show any changes at all. She called for more studies. New trials were carried out, and are still being carried out. To date some 100,000 people have participated in well over 100 clinical studies of pure procaine or the Gerovital mixture. The results of all these studies are confusing and conflicting. This is partly because it is extremely hard to measure general improvements in health by means of clinical studies.

The studies show that, in general, procaine is a mild antidepressant, particularly in relation to the mood, tiredness and depression experienced by the aged. There is a chance that improvements will occur in blood-pressure, body tone, skin texture, hair and in the level of symptoms of the agues of some older people. However, it cannot cure diseases. These changes only occur where procaine is given for several months, and appear to be the same whether pure procaine or the mixture is taken.

It is evident that the effects of procaine are real, and not psychological – many of the studies have used placebos for comparison. But how it works is another story. Procaine is broken down very fast in the body to two components, para-aminobenzoic acid (PABA) and diethyl aminoethanol (DEAE). A few minutes after it is taken internally, only these two substances are left in the body. It is these that have the long term effects, or more specifically, the DEAE portion since PABA is more or less pharmacologically inert. It is known that DEAE enters the brain where it can alter the membranes around brain cells. Although the details are as yet uncertain, the most plausible suggestion so far is that it improves the function of nerve cells, and particularly influences those nerve cells which are in charge of the production of hormones from the brain. Improved hormone production is the consequence, and generates any alterations to skin, hair, arthritis and body symptoms which may occur. In this respect, procaine appears to act not unlike some of the herbs discussed in Chapter 4, although it is a modern chemical. It is not strong, certainly weaker than reasonable quality ginseng, and to some extent ginseng has replaced it as the 'fashionable' restorative. However, many doctors prescribe it all over the world and it is generally recognized as safe by medicine's authorities.

Pick-me-up In Ageing

There are certain drugs prescribed by doctors for confusion, loss of memory and brain damage which can occur in old age. Some of these drugs such as piracetam, metrazol, or procain-imide, act as brain stimulants. Others work by expanding the small blood vessels in the brain, and do provide a certain limited restoration of mental function. However, these drugs are mostly suitable for severe cases and are not normally issued to healthy elderly people. One of these drugs, hydergine, is used extensively in Europe and is prescribed for milder cases. Good reports have emerged concerning its effectiveness. On the other hand, it expands small blood-vessels throughout the body as well as in the brain which may reduce their flexibility in long-term use.

One series of compounds which are used in old age are the classical energy-giving tonics containing glucose or phosphate compounds, for example glycerophosphate. They are sometimes taken in tonic wines. These are only for short term use, and of value in special situations, such as extreme weakness, debility or convalescence. They do not have a long term effect on performance and vitality, but are more like instant foods. They do not affect ageing symptoms or the ageing process. Furthermore, they are of little benefit to health in individuals with a normally functioning metabolism since they add high energy compounds from the outside rather than encouraging the body to make its own, although occasionally they may be needed to 'top-up' the energy stores. It is something of a misnomer to call them tonics.

Tonics should not be confused with classical stimulants such as amphetamine or dexedrine which work directly on the brain as excitants and, unlike the tonics, increase performance and activity, at the cost of sleep and learning ability. They have serious side-effects in the end, leading to greater mental deterioration than there was to start with. They used to be given to old people, especially in institutions, until it was found that on withdrawal of the drug an opposite depressant reaction sets in which may be severe. They are completely useless for health maintenance in older people.

There is a group of mild restorative or anti-depressant drugs which are in widespread use for older people with much more justification. They have an effect not unlike ginseng. In fact, they are closer to ginseng than any other group of Western medicines. These are drugs containing the diethylamino or dimethylamino (DEAE or DMAE) group and include procaine, ('KH3') as we have already noted, DMAE itself ('Deaner') used extensively in the United States as a mild antidepressant especially in the early 1960s, and centrophenoxine or meclofenoxate ('Lucidril') widely described as a geriatric tonic, especially in Europe. These drugs have been studied both in laboratory tests on animals and in trials with people of various ages. In both cases they have been found to have a mildly stimulating effect on the central nervous system. Patients sometimes reported improvements in memory, vitality, alertness, and other psychological attributes, on long-term treatments. They are particularly useful against depression in older people. The mildly stimulating action of DMAE is not accompanied by the side-effects such as insomnia, agitation, excitability or dependence, which are associated with the classical stimulants.

These remedies appear to work through their close chemical relationship with a vital metabolic substance called choline. Choline is taken into the membranes of cells where it becomes part of their innate structure. It is also a precursor of one of the main brain chemical messengers, acetylcholine. DMAE and DEAE are inserted into membranes in addition to choline, where they stabilize their structure and release more choline for its other duty as a part of the brain messenger. The latter accounts for the mental improvements and sense of well-being experienced by many on taking these remedies for lengthy periods.

The membrane stabilization produced by DMAE or DEAE also produces a spin-off. The housekeeping or housecleaning activities of the cells, carried out by little bodies termed 'lysozymes', tend to go somewhat crazy in older tissues. They leave some waste and remove some that should remain. DMAE or DEAE help to stabilize this process. A visible result is that brain cells, which are clogged with age deposit, clean more easily, especially when DMAE is given in the form of centrophenoxime.

DMAE does lengthen the lifespan when fed to mice. An American scientist, Richard Hochschild, added DMAE to mice feed when the mice were already in old age, and found a 50 per cent increase in lifespan compared to a matched group of mice who did not have the DMAE. However, other scientists have been unable to get the same extraordinary result. Hochschild has also been able to extend mouse lifespan using centrophenoxine, although not to the same extent. In this case he is supported by other scientists who

obtained moderate lifespan extensions when feeding centrophenoxine to laboratory mice.

Centrophenoxine and procaine are, for ageing purposes,
preferable to DMAE itself which is mildly stimulating but may
not have the same general restorative effects. Both centrophenoxine and procaine are suitable rejuvenatory substances
for those already past middle age, and the more a person feels
his age, or ages prematurely, the greater the effect of these
materials. Many doctors now recognize their value and
prescribe them freely to their elderly patients. However, it is
doubtful if they are as effective or as strong as ginseng and
eleutherococcus given identical cases. Ginseng has more
unequivocal scientific studies to back up its use, has a more
pervasive effect on body systems and can be taken by younger
people in health maintenance courses, whereas the ethanol-
amine group are not used by younger people in order to
improve health and the lifespan.

7
HELP YOURSELF

The average person in this century ages like a man who crosses a sea and is so careless about his route that he becomes shipwrecked within site of his goal. The ship has been wrecked on the rocks of the degenerative diseases of advanced age: the deterioration of the heart, the blockage of blood vessels, the arthritic stiffening of the joints, and the cancerous growths. While in early life youthful vitality can avoid many diseases, and medicine is capable of curing others, degenerative changes have been allowed to develop insidiously until they inevitably emerge, full-blown and intractable. The degenerative conditions result from the lifestyle, concerning which more useful information can be gleaned in the *Vedas* of 5,000 years ago than the medical textbooks of today. Until these diseases are banished, no further progress can be expected in attaining a ripe old age.

We have discussed in the preceding pages how the environment in which we live, the foods and poisons which we consume and our state of mind have a profound effect on the manner of ageing. It is true that there is a constitutional component to life expectancy, a potential which we receive from our parents. But it is easily overriden by destructive habits. Which habits, then are best? How can we choose and keep to the desirable ones?

Here we encounter major difficulties. For one thing, younger people today have grown up in a more heavily polluted, synthetic, stressful and overmedicated world than the previous generation. They have got off to a rather bad start. At the same time many new health techniques have come into vogue. There lies the second problem. How is one to choose between the courses, health plans, diets, sports, therapies, psychospiritual practices, remedies and personal development schemes? A third problem is psychological. The world we live in is such a turbulent market place. How is one to generate the will and foresight to persist in a chosen way through thick and thin, especially since the benefits may not be immediate?

Ultimately, the art of reaching a healthy old age in our society is self-awareness and self-control, so that a lifestyle can be designed with sensitivity to the formative or destructive agencies inside and outside ourselves. This is more than a counting and measuring of calories, for would not the worry about food intake itself be just another kind of stress? It is more than a fanatical attachment to this or that regime or discipline, for what then is the point of living longer if it is only to become obsessed with a discipline for living longer? It involves the development of a personal path, so that practices such as going for a run every morning, or eating a macrobiotic or vegetarian diet, or retiring to the countryside to cut corn, are carried out with full awareness that this is the appropriate thing to do at the time.

Self-awareness will teach us which procedures are relevant to our constitution, personality, age, environment, type of occupation and so on. For example an agressive, large, hot-blooded man would benefit from a vegetarian diet with mildly tranquilizing herbal teas such as chamomile to help sleep, relaxation and digestion. A thin, timid, and cold person might arrive at the conclusion that he ought to eat meat in reasonable quantities and that an occasional course of ginseng provides a lasting increase in energy and positivity. If your work is physical, you might find that yogic breath control settles the body and opens the mind, while if you work as a clerk, you may discover that you need more dynamic practices such as the martial arts, to unclog the system and sweat-out tension. This could be combined with a Japanese macrobiotic diet since it fits into an overall pre-existing philosophical framework.

In this fashion a path to longevity can be forged, based on

the twin aspects of consciousness – knowledge and self-awareness. Knowledge, of course, can be obtained through courses, books, advice from practitioners and friends, and elements of the culture-based folk wisdom around us. Self-awareness is more difficult to develop. It is based on self-observation combined with sensitivity. On the simplest level this means understanding how the influences of the world around us impinge on our being. How do you feel when you drink coffee or eat sugar? What happens when you do not exercise for a while, or if you do too much exercise too suddenly? What happens when you take this or that remedy, herb or dietary supplement: do you get more or less of any expected problems? What kind of diseases are you prone to anyway and why? Which kinds of experiences do you find most relaxing, and which most stressful? How much stress are you actually receiving and how sensitive are you at detecting it in your mind and in the muscles of your body?

A path arrived at in this way is sure to be absorbed naturally in your lifestyle, without becoming more of a burden than the way of doing things that it was intended to replace. However, it is certainly a path of experience rather than a path of innocence. It is intended for our modern world in which few of us have an arcane and primitive certainty about the right way to live. We are living in an environment which is besieged by ideas which both encourage and discourage mental and physical well being. It so happens that we do not live in the Hunza valley where the sun shines on a harmonious but tough and simple people who may live a very long and healthy life without working at it. We are not Masai tribesmen who have a rock bottom degree of heart defects despite a diet of animal products which we would regard as a cardiovascular catastrophe. The very fact that you are reading this book is an indication that you are not one of those lucky few who get there by intuition alone.

Finding Out

The initial step is to gather more information. There is a selected list of books for further reading at the back of this book. While this book introduces some remedies with special connections to ageing, it does not include remedies to stabilize, purify, support and heal body systems and a thorough knowledge of such home remedies is important. Information is also needed on suitable physical and psycho-physical practices, on dietary procedures and recipes, sources of supply and other people around you who practice similar procedures. Information is needed on psychological development, particularly in relation to relaxation, stress resistance and the development of positivity, self-awareness and self-acceptance.

After obtaining background knowledge, a practitioner should be consulted. This is a valuable and important step, but it sometimes leads to confusion and disappointment where practitioners preaching various systems give contrary advice. For example, a nature-cure practitioner will often recommend salads, uncooked foods and vegetarianism while a Far Eastern therapist trained in macrobiotics or Chinese traditional medicine, might state that such uncooked foods are too 'cooling' and fish is needed. This confusion is inevitable because of the thick undergrowth of separate systems growing up like fresh weeds in untilled fields. The appropriate action would be to take several kinds of advice and select the practitioner who has extensive experience; who is able to tell you most accurately about yourself, your past weaknesses and strengths; and who is able to design for you a dietary and therapeutic regime that feels right for you. Your intuition should tell you that this therapist has advice that fits the 'patient', the time and the place.

Practitioners trained in naturopathy, herbalism and anthroposophy often fit the bill. Some, but by no means all, practitioners in homeopathy or traditional Chinese acupuncture, have the training and experience to work with you on your lifestyle.

Turning from Drugs

Change is the source of benefit, but can also be a potential source of trauma and disruption. Any major alterations in life habits must be introduced slowly and harmoniously, especially in older ages. This particularly applies to food, exercise and drugs.

It is essential to minimize or eliminate the use of strong

drugs wherever possible, even if side effects are not immediately apparent. We have already discussed the severe cost of drug treatment to general health. It is, of course, very tempting to seek short-term relief, and in many cases it might be dangerous not to do so. Yet too often a situation develops in which neither the doctor nor the patient is willing to give up medication despite creeping toxic side-effects. Only when the side-effects themselves become more serious than the original disease, will the doctor make the difficult decision to withdraw the drugs. Drug treatment is therefore mostly a juggling operation between the benefit and the harm of drugs. Indeed, one respected geriatrician reported that 'some of the most dramatic effects of drug therapy in the elderly are achieved not in initiation but in withdrawal (of treatment)'. Once unnecessary drugs are withdrawn, mild, long-term and safe remedies, accompanied by changes in diet and way of life, can begin to take effect.

A word of warning is necessary. Health is elusive and requires a steady and careful approach over a long-term period. Until that is achieved, it is important not to sabotage the doctor's effort without substituting anything in its place. For example, if the doctors give medication which an individual takes only sporadically it makes it impossible for the doctor to treat that person while, without knowledge of the consequences, that person is not treating himself. That is the worst of both worlds and can lead to serious health problems. Refusal to take a cardiac tonic, for example, could be fatal. The correct way of dealing with a situation where it is suspected that medication is unnecessary is to request the doctor to gradually withdraw it, and discuss with him the alternative measures and advice you are taking for the health problem involved. In that way careless and self destructive actions can be avoided.

The Control of Diet

Our earlier discussions on vitamins, supplements and dietary control, can be summarized as follows:

1. Avoid processed, purified, canned, packaged food like the plague. Avoid white sugar, white bread, instant foods and reduce coffee and alcohol. Do not use aluminium pans.

2. Eat sparingly and 'leave the table unsatisfied', is a generally useful rule. Avoid any high protein or high calorie diet.

3. Take in useful supplements in the form of vitamin and mineral-rich foods such as yeasts, wheat germ, seeds, and fruit.

4. Avoid polluted contaminated air and water wherever possible, and attempt to use organically grown produce.

5. Fast occasionally. Any fast of more than two days should be under the guidance of a practitioner.

It is not possible to be more specific, given the individualistic nature of beneficial health programmes. It is usual practice for a naturopathic practitioner to initiate a health maintenance programme with a proper fast or an extended period of limited food, in order to purify the system and remove toxins. This is often aided by blood-purifying herbs.

Care of the Body

When it comes to exercise and breathing even more care is needed to ensure adequate results without suddenly damaging the body. Gradually take more exercise of a rhythmic and non-violent character. The transition must be gradual. Walking, cycling and swimming are beneficial. Yoga or medical gymnastics of the Taoists type even more so. The goal should not be exercise of the muscles, but of the whole body, its blood-vessels, lungs, heart and hormone glands. For this purpose a variety of exercises are recommended, particularly inverse postures (head or shoulder stand) for increasing blood circulation in the brain and preventing neck arthritis, twists and bends to increase spinal suppleness and massage the internal organs, postural correction to maintain strength and balance and delay degenerative changes to the skeleton, chest exercises for the heart and lungs, breath retention and control for calming the mind and improving the efficiency of aeration of the blood.

The Choice of Remedies

It is one thing to give recipes, and quite another to advise the cook when to cook them. The remedies discussed in this book all have their special uses. But a certain amount of trial and error, or serendipity, and of personal taste, will decide who takes what and when.

Assuming that a fairly healthy individual wishes to design a system of self-administration of remedies and supplements to increase his chances of longevity and a healthy old age. He should aim for three things: protection, purification and positive energy. This applies to any adult. However, the emphasis should change with time from protection at younger age to positive energy at older ages. Protection is the realm of the vitamins and minerals we have discussed, C, E, B_3, selenium, sulphur compounds and so on. Purification is the realm of some of the herbs, e.g. peppermint, sage and chamomile, used as mild teas to clean and clear the system. Positive energy largely refers to the ginseng-type plants and the DMAE/DEAE chemicals along with others from various parts of the globe, such as sarasparilla, Brahmi and kava-kava.

Supposing you really do feel your age, that in addition to beneficial health practices you feel that you need something stronger to get you going, or supposing you are recovering from a chronic disease, or a lengthy period of events which have been disastrous to your health. In those situations you should consider a full restoration therapy. This might be a cell-therapy treatment, a period in a natural hospital or residential centre undergoing supervised fasts and internal purifications. It might build a basis for further self-treatment.

At younger ages do not take any of the restorative remedies continuously, unless you need them because of convalescence. There is a danger of the body becoming conditioned to them over a long period so that they do very little good any more. In some cases, as in the overconsumption of ginseng or procaine, mild side-effects may appear. Therefore, take courses of the supplements and restorative remedies and nothing in between. In late middle age and beyond it is possible to take these materials continuously, provided they are clearly the ones that suit you.

When you take any remedy, observe carefully changes which occur in your health and inner state. Add the information to that provided by your adviser. Gradually it will be possible to evolve your own individual 'mix' of remedies which embody the qualities of protection and prevention, purification and energy in the right amounts according to your own individual needs. Whatever you try should be given a chance to work. Herbal remedies are slow and cumulative. The protection of vitamin supplementation rises gradually. Health builds slowly.

Cost and availability also come into the picture. It is useful to buy remedies in bulk which can save a very great deal of money. There are herbal suppliers, growers and importers who supply herbs, and sometimes vitamins in quantity. They can usually be found through societies which support herbs and natural medicine. Vitamins, where possible, should be taken in their natural form, derived from organic sources. Thus vitamin C derived from rose-hips, with added rutin and bioflavonoids to aid absorbtion and metabolism in the body, will be better than pure vitamin C from a chemist, and provided it is bought in bulk, no more expensive. The health-food trade in western countries is now highly sophisticated. There will be many forms of the various herbal and dietary supplemental preparations. It is advisable to read carefully the dosages and contents of all the preparations, make sure you know it is exactly what you want, and obtain it as pure and inexpensive as possible. Very often your health adviser will be able to recommend sources of supply.

It might be argued that a truly healthy person should not take any remedies or supplements at all. Bailey, a well known Victorian writer on longevity states:

> It is not the rich and the great, not those who depend on medicines or the rules of dietitians who become old, but such as use much exercise, are exposed to the fresh air, and whose food is plain and moderate . . .

Did old Parr take remedies? Do the Hunza Valley people? It is true that an absolutely healthy person need not take anything at all. But who is absolutely healthy? Everyone goes through episodes of lower health, of vulnerability or sensitivity, of stresses and shocks. Remedies are necessary on occasions but the healthier you are, the less need you have of them. They then become occasional extra tools to maximize resistance. Even in the Hunza valley they eat a good deal of wild apricot kernels. As we have seen these are the best source of vitamin B_{12}, (amygdalin), which has been claimed to increase resistance to cancer and some other conditions. Rarely is there a society or culture in which even the healthiest of people do not take local herbs, fruit or seeds in order to modify or adjust their bodies to the seasons, the temperature and other changes of environment.

Yet there is no reason to be too dependent or obsessed with remedies. In fact, the use of remedies can very easily lead to a kind of transference of responsibility for health from one's inner resources to external aids. Many people in the West, aided by the health-food industry, might see in remedies a simple solution to problems that go much deeper. It is, after all, much easier to pop a pill in one's mouth, to brew a herb tea, or even to eat special foods, than to confront the source of most ill-health which is one's own mind.

The Economy of Arousal

No book on health can leave out the influence of states of mind. This is particularly the case where ageing is concerned. For during the lifespan mental attitudes become imprinted on the body in the long-term tensions leading to arthritis, stresses pouring out unnecessary hormones and leading to vulnerability and deterioration of the heart and blood-vessels, depression reducing the metabolism and disturbing body rhythms, anxiety ruining the digestion, and all kinds of mental imbalance preventing the discipline of self-care which is a prerequisite of a long life. In old age, attitude and caste of mind are just as important. A person who feels young and alive, and is interested and involved in life, will be more likely to survive. On the other hand, a person who gives up after retirement, who is resigned and lethargic can become submerged in passivity and depression, leading frequently to institutional care and an early demise.

Research into psychological attitudes of the very long-lived indicate that the prime attributes are inner tranquility and self-acceptance. This does not mean that one has to find the wisdom of Solomon in order to attain the age of Methusaleh. Indeed it is often advantageous to be quite simple and uneducated in attaining beneficial inner states. Self-acceptance is most often destroyed by emotional turmoil and emotional immaturity, or by an overactive cerebral cortex leading to a semi-permanent argument with life.

One writer on longevity comments:

'It may be safely doubted whether a single instance can be found of a man of violent and irascible temper. . . who has arrived at a very advanced period of life.'

It is wonderfully easy to state desirable qualities of mind and a lifetime's work to achieve them. There are basically two complementary ways: centrifugally, from the inside outwards, and centripetally, from the outside in. The first is the way of psycho-analysis, of contemplation, prayer, confession, exorcism, counselling and all the other methods of sorting out inner confusions and arriving at a more peaceful co-existence with self. The second method, which we shall briefly explore here, attacks the problem from its manifestations. It involves centreing, quietening and stress reduction techniques. The rationale is that no matter what the source of agitation or confusion, it is possible to let the problems flow on and away without causing psychosomatic disruption.

Some of these stress reduction techniques are widely taught; hypnotherapy to reduce obsessive and compulsive drives, meditation to quiet the mind, relaxation methods to give the body defence systems a rest or autogenic training to provide a systematic 'Western' method for achieving mental and physical peacefulness. It would seem that unless one lives in a harmonious rural environment, with little stress and a clear sanguine and relaxed personality to match, it would be advisable for everyone to develop or learn ways of total relaxation, ways of returning to their own child-like and peaceful centre. Again, different methods can be studied or tried until the right one is found.

One aspect which is common to all these methods is a reduction in arousal. Each of us has an optimum degree of arousal within which we work best. Under-arousal is harmful, leading to atrophy of body defences and under-use of the physiology. Too much arousal means a damaging overuse of body stress-resisting systems which are burdened by excessive watchfulness. This is the most common problem in the modern world, in which the urban population are continually bombarded with noise, television, cars, advertising, telephone, and demands of the multitude of 'flies in the marketplace' as

Nietsche put it. A Swedish study of industrial workers has shown that when they worked for months without a holiday, their adrenal stress hormones could never properly switch off. They suffered from insomnia, perpetual tiredness, poor vitality and psychosomatic disease. After they took a holiday, their adrenal glands recovered the ability to switch off properly and their health improved.

Perhaps the Taoist's greatest secret weapon for longevity was not a remedy at all, but their training in quietism, *wu wei*. This does not mean a cosy insulation from life. Rather, they practiced at attaining *economic arousal*. This means responding to every experience, whether an attack by a man or a bacteria, whether hunger or grief, with precisely that amount of energy needed in the circumstances, not over or under-reacting and allowing the experience to disappear without traces afterwards.

It is walking the thin line between over and under-use. It is naturally impossible to live like a Hunza villager or Taoist recluse, in the middle of Manhattan. Yet a steady approach towards efficient arousal and a calm centre, is something that we can all work for, whether we have instruction or not. It is, I believe, one of the key secrets of a long life. I find it, invariably, in the extremely old and healthy people whom I have met, whatever they eat, wherever they live, and whether or not they have taken any special remedies. It has an important spin-off. Our lives will become more satisfying. It would be a mistake to pay too much attention to longevity and health itself, an attention which is only the mirror of a constant fear of death. It is a trap some ardent prolongevists have fallen into. What after all, do we want to do with the years we have? Efforts to improve health and longevity should arise naturally from the way we live. In this way we might hope to add life to our days as well as days to our life.

BIBLIOGRAPHY

Ageing and Longevity

Mann, J.A. *Secrets of Life Extension,* Harbor Publishing, San Francisco (1980).

Comfort, A. *Ageing: The Biology of Senescence,* Churchill Livingstone, Edinburgh (1980).

Lindsay,R. *The Pursuit of Youth,* Pinnacle. New York (1976).

Hochschil, R. *Gerontologia,* 19 271 (1973).

Rosenfeld, A. *Prolongevity,* Knopf, New York (1976)

Sheehy, G. *Passages,* Dutton, New York (1976).

Beveridge, Ann. *The Road to Shangri-La: My 60,000 Mile Quest for the Secrets of Rejuvenation,* Arlington, U.K. (1979).

Vitamins and Diet and Self-care

Davis, A. *Let's Eat Right to Keep Fit,* Allen & Unwin, London (1979).

Di Cyan, E. *Vitamin E and Aging,* Pyramid, New York (1972).

Gerras, C. (ed) *The Complete Book of Vitamins,* Rodale Press, Aylesbury (1977).

Frank, B.S. and Miele, P. *Dr Frank's No-Aging Diet,* Dell, New York (1976).

Passwater, R.A. *Supernutrition,* Thorsons, Wellingborough (1981).

Stone, I. *The Healing Factor: 'Vitamin C' against Disease,* Grosset and Dunlap, New York, (1972).

Pfeiffer, C.C. *Mental and Elemantal Nutrients,* Keats, Connecticut (1975). Available in U.K. from Thorsons, Wellingborough.
Moyle, A. *Natural Health for the Elderly,* Thorsons, Wellingborough (1975).

Procaine

Bailey, H. *GH3: Will It Keep You Younger Longer?* Bantam, New York (1977).
Aslan, A. *Die Therapiewoche,* 7 14 (1956).

Cell Therapy

Schmid, F. and Stein J. (eds) *Zellforschung und Zelltherapie,* Hans Huber, Bern (1963).
Niehans, P. *Introduction to Cellular Therapy,* Pageant, New York (1960).

Herbs in General

Lucas, R. *Nature's Medicines,* Parker New York (1966).
Kourenoff, P.M. and St. George, G. *Russian Folk Medicine,* W.H. Allen, London (1970).
Mellor, C. *Natural Remedies for Common Ailments,* C.W. Daniel, Saffron Walden (U.K.).
Grieve, M. *A Modern Herbal,* Penguin (1976).

Ginseng and Oriental Remedies

Fulder, S. *About Ginseng,* Thorsons, Wellingborough, (1976).
Fulder, S. *The Root of Being; Ginseng and the Pharmacology of Harmony,* Hutchinsons, London (1980), also entitled, *The Tao of Medicine: Oriental Remedies and the Pharmacology of Harmony* Inner Traditions International, New York, (1982).
Brekhman, I.I. and Dardymov, I.V., *Annual Review Pharmacology* 9, 419 (1969).
Brekhman, I.I. *An Introduction to the Pharmacology of Health,* Pergamon Press, Oxford (1979).
Palos, S. *The Chinese Art of Healing,* Bantam, New York (1972).

Psychological and Psychosomatic Therapies

Simonton, O.C. Mathews-Simonton, S. and Creighton, J.L.,

Getting Well Again Bantam Books, New York (1980).
Benson, H. *The Relaxation Response,* William Morrow, New York (1975).
Pelletier K.R. *Mind as Healer, Mind as Slayer,* Delta, New York (1977).
Wood, E. *Yoga,* Penguin London (1972).
Schultz, J.H. and Luthe W. *Antogenic Training,* New York (1959).

Medicine and Alternative Medicine

Carlson, R.J. *The End of Medicine,* John Wiley, New York and London (1975).
Illich, I. *Medical Nemesis – The Expropriation of Health,* Penguin, U.K. (1976).
Stanway, A. *Alternative Medicine,* Macdonald and Janes, London (1979).
Eagle R. *Alternative Medicine,* Futura, London (1978).
Hastings A.C., Fadiman, J. and Gordon J.S. *Health for the Whole Person* Westview Press, Boulder, Colorado (1980).
Forbes, A. *Try Being Healthy,* Langdon Books, Plymouth (1976).
Fulder, S.J. *The Handbook of Complementary Medicine,* Coronet, Hodder & Stoughton, London (1983).

INDEX